Care Planning in
Mental Health

Dedicated to:

Nigel (RIP)

Care Planning in Mental Health

Promoting Recovery

Second Edition

**Edited by Angela Hall, Michael Wren
and Stephan D. Kirby**

All editors at:
School of Health and Social Care,
Teesside University,
Middlesbrough,
UK

WILEY Blackwell

This edition first published 2013, © 2013 by John Wiley & Sons, Ltd
First editions © 2008 Blackwell Publishing Ltd.

Registered Office
John Wiley & Sons, Ltd, The Atrium, Southern Gate, Chichester, West Sussex, PO19 8SQ, UK

Editorial Offices
9600 Garsington Road, Oxford, OX4 2DQ, UK
111 River Street, Hoboken, NJ 07030–5774, USA

For details of our global editorial offices, for customer services and for information about
how to apply for permission to reuse the copyright material in this book please see our website
at www.wiley.com/wiley-blackwell

Library of Congress Cataloging-in-Publication Data
Care planning in mental health : promoting recovery / edited by Angela Hall, Michael Wren,
Dr. Stephan D. Kirby. – 2nd edition.
        p. ; cm.
    Includes bibliographical references and index.
    ISBN 978-0-470-67186-3 (paperback)
I. Hall, Angela, 1962– editor of compilation. II. Wren, Mike, 1967- editor of compilation.
III. Kirby, Stephan D., editor of compilation.
[DNLM: 1. Mental Health Services. 2. Mental Disorders–rehabilitation.
3. Patient Care Planning. WM 30]
    RC440
    616.89′0231–dc23
                                            2013018016
A catalogue record for this book is available from the British Library.

Wiley also publishes its books in a variety of electronic formats. Some content that appears in print
may not be available in electronic books.

Cover image: iStock © urbancow
Cover design by His and Hers Design, www.hisandhersdesign.co.uk

Set in 10/12.5pt Palatino by SPi Publisher Services, Pondicherry, India

1   2013

Contents

Contributors

Sarah Bonney RMN, Dip (H&SW), BSc (Hons)
Sarah has been a mental health nurse for 24 years in a variety of settings including a community recovery team and a rural community eating disorder team in the NHS Lincolnshire Trust. She currently works at British Columbia Children's Hospital, Canada, within the provincial specialised eating disorder programme.

Jim Campbell MA, RN (Mental Health), Dip (Training & Development)
Jim is a self-employed mental health trainer based in Edinburgh. He is also a researcher, writer and practitioner, specialising in recovery and sexual abuse. He has worked for over 15 years in both healthcare and education and is currently working as a person-centred counsellor in Primary Care. He enjoys writing, publishing in a range of areas and is on the Editorial Collective of Asylum Magazine. He recently coauthored, with Ron Coleman, *Reclaiming Our Lives: A Workbook for Males Who Have Experienced Sexual Abuse*, which draws on the direct experiences of the authors' own recovery journeys. His passion and enthusiasm lies in recovery, giving people hope that change can and will happen.

Charlotte Chisnell BA (Hons), PgCE, Cert (HE)
Charlotte has had a career in Social Work which has spanned over 20 years predominately within safeguarding and youth offending based within Glasgow and the Northeast. Charlotte's last post was with a Youth Offending Team working with persistent young offenders. Her research interests centre around safeguarding, law and mental health issues for young people. Charlotte is also currently undertaking a Masters in Mental Health Law. At present, Charlotte is a Senior Lecturer at the School of Health and Social Care, Teesside University. She is Module Leader for the Social Policy and Law modules on the Social Work BA Degree programme and Module Leader on the Contemporary Issues for Children and Families on the post qualifying Social Work Course.

Sandra Cleminson MA (Creative Writing), Dip (COT)
Sandra is currently a Senior Lecturer in Occupational Therapy at Teesside University. Having worked for 16 years in mental health as an Occupational Therapist, she came into teaching 9 years ago. Her interest in service user perspective has always been central to her work, and during the past 5 years she has been able to include this more directly in teaching sessions by involving service users. Her involvement with Aidan Moesby has allowed both of them to develop a collaborative relationship where they have aimed to promote mental health awareness and the need for service user led therapy. They have presented at conferences and written a journal article together about the way they work and hope this inspires others to do the same. She is passionate about the development of services and professionals that aim to put the person central whilst promoting recovery.

Dr. Mike Fleet BSc, MSc, RMN, RGN, RNT, PgCE, Dip (Thorn), DProf, FHEA
Mike is a Senior Lecturer, at the School of Health and Social Care, Teesside University, and is Module Leader for several programmes in Recovery and Psychosocial Interventions. He is the Field Leader for Pre-registration Mental Health Nursing and leads a recovery-focused module on promoting positive outcomes for people affected by mental health issues. Mike's doctoral research involved a critical enquiry into the concept of care and recovery on a Psychiatric Intensive Care Unit. Before entering the field of lecturing, Mike was Clinical Nurse Specialist with the South West London and St. George's Hospital Mental Health NHS Trust's Assertive Community Treatment Team.

Scott Godfrey MA (Ed), PgCE (HE), BSc (Hons) Nursing, ADNS, RN
Scott qualified as a registered nurse in 2001 from Teesside University. His passion for emergency care, and trauma management, resulted in him perusing a career within the Emergency Department (ED). Scott currently works as a Senior Lecturer at Teesside University and has worked in higher education for the past 6 years. In 2011, Scott completed an MA in Education and developed a particular interest in reflective writing. His academic responsibilities include pre- and postregistration module leadership, he is a field leader for Adult Nursing and is currently working as an External Examiner for Essex University. Scott also has a strong interest in acute and emergency care and in nursing education.

Angela Hall MA, BSc (Hons), RMN, RGN, RNT, EdD Student (Durham) (co-editor)
Angela has been qualified as a Mental Health Nurse for 30 years and has been in nursing education for the past 20 years. Her main experience was as a Community Psychiatric Nurse working with adults and older people within a primary care setting and then later within a Community Mental Health Team. She became a nurse educator in 1992, and her MA thesis was

in Humanistic Counselling. Her current interests are in human potential, recovery and caring.

Natalie Iley BSc (Hons), Cert (AdvEd), RNLD, RSW

Natalie originally worked with adults experiencing challenging behaviour in a community-based setting and has continued to work alongside adults with learning disabilities within a variety of settings for 5 years. She completed her BSc (Hons) Social Work and Learning Disabilities Nursing and remains committed to the philosophies of obtaining her dual qualification, choosing to pursue a career in social work within integrated teams. Natalie's current role is as a Registered Social Worker for Adults, Older People and Safeguarding and spans nearly 5 years. She is currently working closely as a Practice Educator with Teesside University to support students and their transition to becoming a qualified Social Work Practitioner. Natalie's interests include supporting people with learning disabilities to achieve realistic goals through meaningful activities and working with older people to maintain and achieve independence within their own local communities.

Dr. Stephan D. Kirby PhD, MSc, PgCE (L&T), UCPPD (L&T), Dip MDO, RMN (co-editor)

Steve is a son, father, grandfather and occasional user of mental health services (as well as a Registered Mental Nurse, a Senior Lecturer and Buddhist Practitioner – must try harder!!). Currently, he is a Senior Lecturer (Forensic Mental Health) in the School of Health and Social Care at Teesside University. He has over three decades of working with people with mental health (and associated) problems, the largest part being within Forensic Mental Health Services. The research for his PhD (in 2010) explored 'What is the meaning of segregation for prisoners'. He has researched and published extensively on a range of mental health and forensic mental health matters and was a coeditor of *Mental Health Nursing: Competencies for Practice* published by Palgrave in 2004 as well coeditor of the first edition of this text *Care Planning in Mental Health: Promoting Recovery*.

Devon Marston

Devon is musician, actor and mental health campaigner. His musical career began with lovers rock band 'the Investigators'. He also acted on the West End stage. Following an episode of mental ill health, he worked to found Sound Minds, an arts and mental health charity. He now helps facilitate music and drama sessions and is a member of the award-winning reggae band 'the Channel One Band' and Chair of the charity's trustees. Devon feels strongly about speaking out on mental health issues and has a national media profile, with appearances on news and current affairs programmes such as BBC2's *Newsnight*; Radio 4's *Today*; Radio 5 *Live* and Channel 4 *News* as well as working with Comic Relief on the *Time to Change* TV campaign. Devon was nominated for a Mental Health Media Award in 2002.

Gordon J. Mitchell RN, Dip Nursing (Lond); BSc (Hons) Nursing Science, PgD (L&T), MA (Advanced Nursing Practice)
Gordon is currently Principal Lecturer for Mental Health and the Course Director for IAPT Programmes in the School of Health and Social Care at Teesside University. The majority of his clinical experience has been gathered in acute mental health units, culminating finally in the opening of a new acute unit in North Durham as a Charge Nurse. Since moving into education, he has worked in a number of areas, including the training of Healthcare Assistants and qualified staff through CPD provision, becoming Pathway Leader for preregistration Mental Health Nursing and finally Principal Lecturer. He is also an NMC Reviewer for preregistration Mental Health Nursing programmes. He became the Course Director for Improving Access to Psychological Therapies programmes when Teesside University was successful in securing the training for qualified CBT therapists and Psychological Wellbeing Practitioners with both programmes receiving accreditation with relevant professional bodies. He has previously written book chapters on the law and presented papers at regional and national conferences.

Aidan Moesby MA (Art and Psychotherapy) Artist, Writer, Facilitator, TrainerTeesside University, Launchpad Newcastle, The Art House (Wakefield)
As a socially engaged artist working primarily with text, Moesby explores relationships between people and places. He is intrigued by rituals and personal myth – repetitive and mundane. From these interactions, he produces responsive interventions, including site-specific installations for venues including spaces for health and contemporary art. He works extensively in Arts and Health, particularly around Mental Health. He works with a variety of health and cultural organisations around wider issues of Disability and Equality in development, training and facilitating. http://aidanmoesby.co.uk/

Teresa Moore RMN, RN, MA (Hons) Health Service Management
Teresa is a Senior Lecturer in Mental Health at the School of Health & Social Care, Teesside University. She is Module Leader for Pre-registration Mental Health Nursing Skills for students in the second year of the Programme, promoting holistic nursing care for those with mental illness. Prior to her post with Teesside University, she worked as a Lecturer/Practitioner in Mental Health, in a joint post with East London and the City NHS Mental Health Trust and City University. Her interest in the complex physical and mental health needs of the older adult, particularly in the area of dementia nursing, continues.

Donna Piper MSc, BA (Hons), PgCE (L&THE), Cert. Ed, Dip (Early Years)
Donna is a Senior Lecturer at the School of Health and Social Care, Teesside University. She is module leader for Advanced Research in Social Work and final year dissertation projects, including care coordinator spanning years 1 to 4 on the BA (Hons) Social Work degree programme. Donna is also the Admissions Tutor for the Social Work programme. She has pursued a career spanning over 19 years predominantly with young people, children and their families in specialist teams. Her research interests are driven by a passion for working with children/young people, societal inequalities, substance use and offending. Her last post was with a 'Leaving Care' Team working with 'Looked After Children/Young People'.

Dr. Theo Stickley Associate Professor of Mental Health – University of Nottingham
Theo is a Mental Health Nurse and also trained as a counsellor. He leads the MSc in Recovery and Social Inclusion at Nottingham and has also researched these subjects. His research interests are mainly focused on the arts and mental health and his book *Qualitative Research in Arts and Mental Health* offers a unique perspective on this specialist subject. When he is not thinking about work, Theo is a keen gardener and motorcyclist and is a member of the Nottingham Society of Artists.

Julie Wardell MA, BA (Hons), DipSW, Dip (Counselling)
Julie is a qualified Social Worker and Practice Educator. She has worked in children's services, young people's services and adult's services and in the field of substance misuse for 18 years. She is currently the Manager of the Addictive Behaviours Service in Stockton, employed by Tees, Esk and Wear Valleys NHS Foundation Trust. Julie's teams have won awards for Quality Improvement, Working in Partnership with other agencies and tackling stigma and promoting social inclusion. Her accolades include being highlighted for delivering 'innovative' services by *Community Care Magazine* and *Alcohol Concern*.

Jenny Weinstein
Jenny is an Independent Consultant, writer and researcher in health and social care and an honorary lecturer at Kingston University. Her experience spans practice, teaching and development in the statutory, voluntary and university sectors. In her current role as Chair of the Local Involvement Network/HealthWatch, Jenny campaigns alongside service users, carers and community groups for improvements in health and social care services with a particular interest in mental health and coproduction initiatives. Recent research and publication activities, undertaken in collaboration with service users and carers, have focused on mental health service user involvement, recovery and personalisation.

Mike Wren BA (Ed), MA (Ed), CertEd, CSS, FAETC, CMS, DMS, MCIM, RSW, RMCSW (co-editor)

Mike has worked in a variety of social work positions spanning more than 19 years, including at senior management level in relation to older people, children and learning disability community-based services. Mike's career has predominantly involved direct contact with children in schools and with special educational needs. His interests include transitions from childhood to adulthood, development of supported living schemes for people with learning disabilities and exploring adult placement provisions for older people to enable individuals to live within their own local communities. Mike joined Teesside University in July 2004 and took up the position of Course Coordinator for BSc (Hons) Social Work & Mental Health Nursing & Social Work & Learning Disability Nursing programmes. In 2010, he became Programme Leader for the BA (Hons) Social Work programme, where he continues to develop his passion for encouraging collegiate approaches toward integrated collaborative working, interprofessional education and practice-based learning opportunities with a wide range of partners from practice.

Dr. Nicola Wright PhD, MA

Research Fellow – Collaboration for Leadership in Applied Health Research and Care (CLAHRC) Nottinghamshire

Nicola Wright is a registered mental health nurse and has worked clinically in both inpatient and community mental health before completing an Economic and Social Research Council-funded MA in Research Methods (2005) and PhD in Nursing Studies in 2009. Since completing her PhD, Nicola has worked in the School of Psychology at the University of Birmingham on a multisite randomised control trial of Joint Crisis Plans for people with Psychosis. She is currently a Research Fellow at the Collaboration for Leadership in Applied Health Research and Care – Nottinghamshire, Derbyshire and Lincolnshire (CLAHRC-NDL).

Chapter 1

Introduction: The Emergence of Recovery as a Key Concept

Stephan D. Kirby, Angela Hall and Mike Wren

Teesside University, UK

> *We shall never cease from exploration. And the end of all our exploring*
> *Will be to arrive where we started. And know the place for the first time*
> T.S. Eliot (Little Gidding)

At the end of the first edition, we left you with two rhetorical questions that arose as a consequence of producing that text:

> *How different would services look if their primary focus was to enable people to use and develop their skills, make the most of their assets and pursue their aspirations?,*

and

> *Would this not change, for the better, the experience of using services, and the relationship between workers, and those whom we serve?* (Repper & Perkins, 2003:11)

In this second edition, we hope to address these questions and in doing so raise your awareness of wider issues and concepts so that you are better informed to decide if you want to be agents of and for the organisation or champions of future change.

Building upon the strengths of our previous book (still available at all good book sellers, Blackwell Publishing website and Amazon), this current text utilises a more conceptual and person-focused approach that will enable the reader to plan for the future, and to challenge political, medical, social and professional identity issues. It is worth pointing out that even though this is a second edition, we have not simply, as is traditional, taken

Care Planning in Mental Health: Promoting Recovery, Second Edition.
Edited by Angela Hall, Michael Wren and Stephan D. Kirby.
© 2013 John Wiley & Sons, Ltd. Published 2013 by John Wiley & Sons, Ltd.

the original chapters and updated them; rather, we have preferred to reflect the developments and advances in mental health care and recovery. We felt it was important that the book reflected the notion that care planning is not simply APIE; rather, it is a move from a professional model focus to the active promotion of the person and their individually constructed narrative. So by engaging with the person's resilience, reserves and inner resources, we are able to focus recovery work around the individual, their story, hopes, dreams, skills and strengths rather than the symptoms of their mental distress (Saleebey, 2009). To address this paradigm shift, our stance within this text openly acknowledges, introduces and applies a variety of differing concepts and ideas underpinning the fact that we best serve people on their journey to recovery by collaborating with them (White & Epstein, 1990).

The reader will find (and we make no apologies for this) that there is no – or very little – explicit mention of APIE as a care-planning process. Whilst this is inherent within the text, it is not the primary focus of this work; rather, we are offering the reader insights into ways of approaching and understanding an alternative underpinning philosophy when implementing care planning in mental health. The structures of Care Planning are well documented and established within the delivery of mental health care; what we hope the reader will gain from this text is a more enlightened and person-focused way of approaching the activities involved in planning collaborative, interprofessional and person-centred care that gives the person with the mental health problem the hope, optimism and opportunity to express their own desires, aspirations and potential that will enhance their journey on the road to recovery.

In the first edition, we attempted to address the issues around recovery as a concept and its application within the care-planning process. However, we were directed by the traditional and dominant frameworks that pervade mental health: such as Care Programme Approach (CPA), a range of 'new' legislations (e.g., the then proposed amendment of the Mental Health Act 1983 (DoH, 1983), the influences of numerous medical model-focused clinical practice guidelines and not forgetting the APIE of the prescriptive Nursing Process. The dominant culture within mental health has prevented professionals from challenging and progressing recovery-focused practice and has made them into (despite their good intentions and desires) passive recipients of the status quo which is shrouded in new terminology and contemporary rhetoric. They become afraid to deviate from this to embrace the recovery concepts as these are often questioned by the organisation as they are not seen to be part of the corporate vision and identity, which is invariably based upon financial requirements and popular trends with no thought for the people receiving and centrally involved in the care. In policy terms, mental health needs to be more concerned with health and wellbeing as well as providing direct support to people to enable them to function as full citizens in their communities (DoH, 2007). 'Increasingly services aim to go beyond traditional clinical care and help patients back into mainstream society, redefining recovery to incorporate quality of life – a job – a decent place to live – friends and a social life' (Appleby, 2007).

We are conscious that there have been major changes in mental health in the years between these two editions. These encompass a refocusing of organisational structure, culture and delivery models. We have continued to see legislative documents and dictates published as well as the further move into community care and, in some cases, even the rebirth and refocus of inpatient provision. Most importantly is the drive, through education and into services, towards the further promotion of the recipient of mental health services being accepted as human beings and equal partners.

This has reawakened the emphasis on 'The Person' (their essence, attributes, uniqueness and individuality and all the factors that exert an influence on personhood) and the hopeful demise of interchangeable labels of stigma, discrimination and depersonalisation. It is obvious that there are, and will be, difficulties and resistances to the professional's acceptance and adoption of these 'new' (though not really new, just old ideas rebranded and repackaged) ways of perceiving the new mental health landscape. There are resistors from all sides, the need to meet organisational targets (the ubiquitous audits and quotas which appear to (and indeed *do*) drive and underpin service provision), both the personal and organisational paranoia of litigation that appears to underpin service delivery today; and the need to have every meeting with the person with the mental health problem; every action; assessment; intervention and interaction recorded and rated on a sliding scale of risk and the appropriate risk management strategies created accordingly. There are ever-decreasing timescales and ever-increasing caseloads that services have to contend with, as well as the change in funding and the move towards a market-led provision with GP fund holding imminent; resistance from individuals and organisations abound. Organisations are being driven by 'New Managerialism' (Hafford-Letchfield, 2009) which relies on targets and outcome-driven agendas and where the illusion of being an involved customer is created and maintained, but in reality, people are merely a commodity of the market place. Recovery provides a new rationale for mental health services and has implications for the design and operation of mental health services and partnerships between health, social services and third-sector organisations (Shepherd *et al.*, 2008).

Whilst in the latter half of the last century, recovery was thought to be an alien concept (Coleman, 1999), it is now firmly on agendas; indeed, it *is* the agenda. Work started by Romme and Escher in their seminal work with voice hearers started a paradigm shift (Romme & Escher, 1993) and it is up to everybody to continue that work until the shift is complete. The Hearing Voices Network, informed by this work of Romme and Escher, works positively with people's experiences of hearing voices (Rogers & Pilgrim, 2010). Rather than trying to obliterate the voices, as a traditional symptom-based approach might do, this user-led initiative attributes meaning to voice hearing. This offers alternative means of coping with voices that may at times cause their recipients distress. Recovery as an idea, a concept and a care focus has now come of age and its importance has been recognised and acknowledged and it provides a new rationale for mental health services (Shepherd *et al.*, 2008). It is based on the notions of self-determination and self-management and emphasises the importance of 'hope' in sustaining motivation (Shepherd *et al.*, 2008). It has become the key principle underlying mental health services across the world, for example, New Zealand (Mental Health Commission, 1998), the United States (Department of Health and Human Services, 2003), Australia (Australian Government, 2003), Ireland (Mental Health Commission, 2005), Scotland (Scotland Government, 2006) and in England (DoH, 2001, 2006, 2007).

Ron Coleman (Coleman, 1999) tells us that there is a common joke amongst people with mental health problems that they all understand, 'What is the difference between God and a Psychiatrist? Answer: God does not think he is a Psychiatrist'. He continues that there is another major difference between God and Psychiatrists: while 'God created the world in 7 days, a Psychiatrist can change a person's in little under an hour' (Coleman, 1999:7). It is no surprise therefore that the road to recovery is difficult and fraught with dangers and traumas, but the road to illness is surprisingly easy – far too easy (Coleman, 1999:7).

It must be pointed out though that this somewhat scathing attitude towards psychiatry and psychiatrists was taken from a number of years earlier in Ron's career towards 'product champion and leader' for voice hearing and trainer for voice hearers. This was a period when clear, distinct lines of battle were drawn between professionals and purveyors of psychiatry and the population that were deemed to be in need, usually against their free will and without consultation, of such disempowering actions. However, as years have passed and with the advent of mental health, so has the culture and climate of recovery. The culture and infantilising nature of psychiatry is diminishing, and partnership working and engagement and empowerment from a recovery framework is growing. Ron and many of his contemporaries now collaborate closely with psychiatrists; indeed, some of his working partners and trainees are psychiatrists. Traditionally, the medical model has served as a means of deflecting attention away from the person and their lived experience(s). None of this is a condemnation of the medical model and psychiatry (as opposed to mental health) per se, but acknowledges the fact that there are limitations to this particular way of representing the experience(s) and problems of living for the person with mental health problems (Barker, 2001). Nor does it, or should it, promote the exclusion of the medical model from the mental health care arena or from the delivery of a person-focused approach to mental health care recovery. Rather, it has its place as does every other approach and discourse; there are times when paternalistic decision making has to occur without the person's involvement and for their best interest. Similarly, there are times, as the person progresses through the phases of recovery, where this approach has to take a back seat and allow the more person-centred, empowering and self-management approach to occur. One that affords the person more growth opportunities towards, and along, an empowering, person-centred approach to recovery within mental health recovery.

But what is recovery? It has been said (Coleman, 1999) that professionals define recovery as maintaining a person in a stable condition, regardless of issues such as adverse effects of medication or even the expressed wish of the person. However, from the person experiencing the mental health problems, recovery is a personal construct, one that is defined by the person themselves, based upon their own experiences and resources. Importantly, the essence of clinical recovery is based upon the premise that clinical recovery occurs because of the effectiveness of the clinical treatment. It is this aspect of recovery, effective (person-centred) treatment that this book is hoping to capture and promote. Recovery is also seen (Anthony, 1993) to be '…a deeply personal, unique process of changing one's attitudes, values, feelings, goals and/or roles…a way of living a satisfying, hopeful and contributing life even with the limitations caused by the illness…the development of new meaning and purpose in one's life as one grows beyond the catastrophic effects of mental illness' (p. 17).

Shepherd *et al.* (2008) offer what they propose to be the key themes of recovery, these being:

1) **Agency** – gaining a sense of control over one's life and one's illness. Finding personal meaning – an identity which incorporates illness, but retains a positive sense of self;
2) **Opportunity** – building a life beyond illness. Using nonmental health agencies, informal supports and natural social networks to achieve integration and social inclusion;
3) **Hope** – believing that one can still pursue one's own hopes and dreams, even with the continuing presence of illness. Not settling for less, that is, the reduced expectations of others.

(Shepherd *et al.*, 2008)

These three overarching themes of recovery were taken on board by the Devon Recovery Group and resulted in the following Principles of Recovery (see Box 1.1). This resulting set of principles (Davidson, 2008) clearly demonstrates an active collaboration of the mutual roles, responsibilities and resources which aim to promote the person, their experience(s) of mental health problems and also reflect a desire and drive to capture the essence of their recovery. These are seen, by the editors, as being key concepts of 'making recovery a reality' (to borrow a phrase from the Sainsbury Centre) and through which we discover the person, their life and celebrate their diversity for, and opportunities to, change. These principles were the inspiration behind, and also formed the underlying belief system for, the development of this text.

Box 1.1   The principles of recovery.

- Recovery is about building a meaningful and satisfying life, as defined by the person themselves, whether or not there are ongoing or recurring symptoms or problems;
- Recovery represents a movement away from pathology, illness and symptoms to health, strengths and wellness;
- Hope is central to recovery and can be enhanced by each person seeing how they can have more active control over their lives ('agency') and by seeing how others have found a way forward;
- Self-management is encouraged and facilitated. The processes of self-management are similar, but what works may be very different for each individual. No 'one size fits all';
- The helping relationship between clinicians and patients moves away from being expert/patient to being 'coaches' or 'partners' on a journey of discovery. Clinicians are there to be 'on tap, not on top';
- People do not recover in isolation. Recovery is closely associated with social inclusion and being able to take on meaningful and satisfying social roles within local communities, rather than in segregated services;
- Recovery is about discovering – or rediscovering – a sense of personal identity, separate from illness or disability;
- The language used and the stories and meanings that are constructed have great significance as mediators of the recovery process. These shared meanings either support a sense of hope and possibility, or invite pessimism and chronicity;
- The development of recovery-based services emphasises the personal qualities of staff as much as their formal qualifications. It seeks to cultivate their capacity for hope, creativity, care, compassion, realism and resilience;
- Family and other supporters are often crucial to recovery and they should be included as partners wherever possible. However, peer support is central for many people in their recovery.

(Davidson, 2008; Shepherd *et al.*, 2008)

One of the central and primary principles of recovery is the notion that it does not necessarily mean cure (clinical recovery); rather, it acknowledges the unique journey a person goes through when building a life beyond mental illness (social recovery) (Shepherd *et al.*, 2008). People have to come to terms with the trauma that the occurrence of mental health symptoms can have on their lives and incorporate these experiences into a new sense of personal identity (Larsen, 2004).

Such traumas can only be resolved if the person can discover – or rediscover – their sense of, and ability to action, personal control (agency) and thus gain a belief in the future (hope); and without hope, (re)building lives cannot begin. Recovery is about this process and the *quality* of this experience is central (Shepherd *et al.*, 2008). The power of, and responsibility for, recovery lies within us – all *users*, professionals and carers – and this can only be achieved by working together, by talking and listening to each other. This can only be done by a paradigm shift from the dominant biological reductionism to one of personal and societal development (Coleman, 1999). This road to self-discovery starts when you look at your own life and how events outside have affected you this includes family, friends, traumatic experiences and life events and how you feel about the things that have happened. A turning point for many people in recovery can be taking the first steps to dealing with feelings of guilt and inadequacy for something you probably have little or no control over. Recovery should follow the premise that professionals should be on tap; not on top (Repper & Perkins, 2003).

Recovery is applicable and appropriate to anyone who experiences a significant mental health problem at any age as well as applied in specialist areas such as forensic mental health services, CAMH Services and Drug and Alcohol Services, and management relies heavily on the provision of information and self-management in addition to treatment and symptom control (Shepherd *et al.*, 2008). Recovery is our common goal, and it is now achievable, so we should not lose the moment for we need to work together to make it happen, and we need to put our past (professional) differences behind us to let us go forward towards recovery (Coleman, 1999).

Many of the ideas underpinning the recovery philosophy are not new (Shepherd *et al.*, 2008). They come from the consumer/survivor movement of the 1980s and 1990s which ran along the lines of self-help, empowerment and advocacy. This was the basis of challenging traditional notions of professional power and expertise which pervaded mental health services (and arguably still do) (Shepherd *et al.*, 2008). These ideas themselves have their roots in the Civil Rights movements of the 1960s and 1970s in the US and in self-help and politically motivated groups such as Mad Pride, Survivor's Speak Out and The Lunatic Liberation Front. From this patients were beginning to be seen, and see themselves, as victims and then survivors of mental health – a notion equitable to those people who survived the concentration camps. Between 1970 and 1990, mental health survivor activity in the UK saw a range of user-led organisations arguing either for the abolition of psychiatry or for its radical reform. These included the 'BNAP' (British Network of Alternatives to Psychiatry), 'PROMPT' (Protection of the Rights of Mental Patients in Therapy) and 'CAPO' (Campaign Against Psychiatric Oppression) (Rogers & Pilgrim, 2010). However, the current recovery movement and frameworks, supported and adopted as they are by a wider range of participants (professionals and users, groups and official bodies), no longer have the political undercurrents of the earlier movements (Shepherd *et al.*, 2008).

There are continuous and consistent concerns that recovery in mental health is being, indeed already has been, hijacked by professionals and that they are rebranding it into a technology, a science, absorbing it into the academic domain and in doing so making it their own. Recovery is now perceived to be a term that is used, possibly indiscriminately, by professionals to represent a panacea of all mental woes; the new 'holism'. The term recovery is used in different contexts by both people with mental health problems and mental health professionals. As recovery ideas have been devised by, and for, patients to describe their individual experiences of their mental health, professionals need to be aware that accusations may be levelled at them for taking over the concept of recovery. There are product champions from both sides who continue to publish around and promote recovery. Despite national policies and frameworks (Shepherd *et al.*, 2008) from a number of diverse organisations, the mental health system continues to be patriarchal and bureaucratic, and ever increasingly so as the years progress and with each subsequent 'development and improvement'.

For recovery to become a reality, professionals need to fully understand the concept of recovery and what it means from a patient perspective so that they can work with the person in the recovery process (Shepherd *et al.*, 2008). Mental health professionals should challenge their own, as well as each other's, negative assumptions and detrimental communications and interactions and strive towards positive attitudes and attributes, because until a sound, collaborative rapport is formed, it is not possible to facilitate a psychoeducational approach. Through the continued usage and promotion of this conceptual shift, one that is mutually beneficial and dynamic and within the framework of interprofessional (partnership) working, the realities of emancipation and empowerment will continue to enable people to no longer 'just exist' but to now 'thrive' in contemporary mental health.

Before we introduce the individual chapters, we would like to offer a quick word on terminology. Language in mental health is a constant site of debate and struggle (Barnes & Bowl, 2001). Not all people with mental health problems reject the notion of 'mental illness', although some do consider the notion of 'illness' an inappropriate and outdated manner of understanding and describing their distress. Similarly, others reject the label 'service user', because of an implication of active engagement with services which does not match their experiences of mental health. 'Consumer' is a term associated with the market and business domains. Others have adopted the terms 'victims' or 'survivor' to portray either a negative or positive image of people in distress and people whose experiences differ from, or who dissent from, society's norms (Barnes & Bowl, 2001). To this end in this text, the reader will find a number of differing terms used throughout the chapters by the differing authors. These are not necessarily those that would have been chosen by the editors, nor by the individual authors themselves; rather, they are used to describe, in a generic, easily conceptualised, widely used and conventional manner, the person who has mental health problems and who engages (or comes into contact) with mental health services. Throughout the editors' individual and combined chapters, they have chosen the term 'person with the mental health problem' – or some derivative – while other authors have gone for the easily understood and conceptualised term of 'patient'; neither – or all – is necessarily always correct or appropriate. The debate regarding a correct term that appropriately describes a person with mental health problems continues, which is why we have chosen to use this term as it is the nearest we can find to a term; a 'label' that does not (hopefully) become a source of discrimination or negativity thus social control and stigma. Even by using a 'soft' term like 'person with mental health problems/person with experiences' is, in itself, a form of labelling; so we are as guilty as anybody of forcing people into categories. Indeed, why do we have to have a nomenclature, a label or some different way of talking about people; surely, they are just 'people' like you and I.

The individual chapters (as summarised in the following text) are grouped into three sections which we believe capture the essence of recovery: 'Survive', 'Manage' and 'Thrive'.

According to Kaplan (1964), when people experience and respond to distress they start to make sense of this; to explain it and to understand it, in essence to survive – despite the difficulties that are happening to them. This starts by people acknowledging they have a problem and seeking assistance wherever they can (or, in some cases, have assistance thrust upon them). Kaplan devised a framework of preventative psychiatry where the person passes through three distinct phases: primary, secondary and tertiary. This moved the person from a point of psychological distress, through diagnosis and treatment to long-term disability. Devised as this was in the 1960s, the recovery model or focus did not exist; indeed, mental health services were exclusively institutional. Hence, Kaplan's model was a reflection of its times. As we moved away from the Institutional Model of mental health, community care has allowed us to see and utilise a more recovery focus to care delivery and services.

Our framework and understanding of the domains of 'Survive', 'Manage' and 'Thrive' reflects, somewhat, Kaplan's (1964) 'Primary', 'Secondary' and 'Tertiary' approach to preventative psychiatry. However, he defined tertiary as a long-term (institutional) care approach for people who had acquired chronicity and were thus engaging on a long-term basis with (institutional) mental health services. We have brought this up to date, and use the domain of 'Thrive' to explain a situation where the person does not seek nor accept chronicity and long-term institutional care. Rather, they seek ongoing recovery and ownership of their illness to a point where they are functioning within a social world to the best of their abilities and skills and continue to learn more about, and engage with, their symptomologies and pathologies, that is, recovery. To enable this to happen, we need, in practical and dynamic ways, to change the 'Manage' aspect of this, that is, the culture and the mindset and practices of people within the organisations, services and cultures. We need to continue to encourage and adopt more interprofessional working activities that include as an equal partner the person with the mental illness.

Our model (and further explanation of the domains of 'Strive', 'Manage' and 'Thrive' and how they interconnect and influence each other) can be found in Chapter 14 and is a visual representation of the amalgamation of all our thoughts and ideas that have driven the development of this text as well as the learning and awareness raising we wished the reader to engage with. It is an amalgamation of Watkins (2001), Kirby (2001) and Kirby & Cross (2002), and we feel this captures the essence of recovery within contemporary, interprofessional, person-centred mental health care.

The chapters

Chapter 2: Experiencing recovery
(Aidan Moesby and Sandra Cleminson)

Through sharing his experiences as a recipient of mental health services, Aidan shares with us the ups and downs, his good and the bad experiences on the road to recovery from a major mental health issue. Through this autobiographical exploration, he offers some clear messages regarding service provision by identifying what made a good, proactive, recovery-focused service and what did not. He clearly shows that effective and wide-ranging support throughout the recovery journey is essential to successful outcomes. This narrative highlights how services can and should meet the needs of the people that need them. It clearly shows that for mental health services to support recovery, they should be tailor-made to the individual and be in the form of what is required on a spectrum of support which is accessible, prevents relapse, empowers and is flexible to need, whilst fostering independence and self-reliance through the use of a model of interprofessional working and recovery.

Chapter 3: Recovery as a framework for care planning
(Jim Campbell, Theo Stickley, Sarah Bonney and Nicola Wright)

In this chapter, Jim and colleagues show how the environment of care that is provided by the mental health professional needs to be supportive and facilitative so that life has meaning for the person with mental health problems. This chapter offers guidance for mental health practitioners to enable them to provide successful recovery-focused mental health care through frameworks for planning care. By drawing on the Sainsbury Centre for Mental Health's Framework for Organisational Change, they show how mental health services need to, and could, change to encompass the concept of recovery. They discuss its values and principles which provide a foundation for more meaningful mental health care, drawing on practical applications and examples from around the world. This chapter then, drawing on literature reviews, offers a number of themes that constitute effective individual recovery and shows how recovery should and could be the norm and how it is a move away from the medical definitions of mental illness to the social construction of recovery; it *can* be normal to be different.

Chapter 4: Discovering the person
(Angela Hall and Donna Piper)

Angela and Donna are asking the salient question of 'do we ever really know anybody' as we only let people see certain aspects of ourselves and our worlds. This is particularly true when a person is going through the turmoil of a crisis in their mental health problems. They propose that effective, recovery-focused assessment can allow professionals come to know people in a more meaningful, less medicalised way. They demonstrate that the use of the term 'assessment' has implications of medicalisation, categorisation and making judgements through the use of structured or outcome-focused tools, which compartmentalise the individual, and how we need to focus this process more on learning about the person with the mental health problems, about their lives, their experiences, their abilities and limitations – the need to capture the richer narratives and discourses. They leave the reader with a very powerful message that we need to really look, not just see, and that we need to listen, and not just hear.

Chapter 5: Parity of esteem
(Mike Wren and Natalie Iley)

Mike and Natalie discuss essential lifestyle planning, which is based on the experiences derived from the person experiencing mental health problems, and go on to discuss the concept of parity of esteem, and how this can reclaim a person's sense of recovery. They introduce the concept, and usage, of 'recovery brokers' who would promote independent functioning with greater credence being given to the personal narrative of the person with mental health problems. They show how this would be underpinned and guided by effective communication, collaboration and coordination. If the development of personal parity of esteem is successful, then the person with the mental health problems would experience 'survivors pride' and have more beneficial experiences and outcomes on their road to recovery.

Chapter 6: Holistic care: physical health, mental health and social factors
(Teresa Moore and Scott Godfrey)

The term 'wellbeing' refers to the achievement of a positive physical, social and mental state as opposed to the absence of mental illness or disease. It is with this premise that Teresa and Scott demonstrate the complex interface of holistic (mental and physical) health care. They clearly show that all forms of mental illness are at increased risk of physical illness and as a consequence can expect a considerably shortened life span as a direct result of mental illness. They also state that as a result of their mental health problems, people are also less likely to access public health initiatives including health screening making early disease detection or intervention less likely. By improving physical health and life expectancy, better educational achievement and employment rates and productivity, reduced antisocial behaviour and criminality and reduced levels of risky behaviours including smoking and alcohol and substance misuse, we can achieve this status of wellbeing for people with mental health problems. It is obvious that any mental health recovery without the inclusion of this holistic dynamism is not complete nor is true to our collaborative partners in care.

Chapter 7: Strengths and diversities: a substance misuse perspective
(Julie Wardell)

By opening her chapter with a very pertinent question, Julie tells us that this is the question asked by anyone interested in the effective promotion of recovery for people who misuse substances (but equally applicable to people with mental health problems). She goes on (while focusing on the Substance Misusing population) to untangle the complex debates regarding the safest and most successful routes to improving an individual's life chances and realising their potential. This chapter then explores ways of working with individuals to promote recovery, such as strengths-based and motivational change practice as well as further identifying and exploring the importance of working with individuals in a person-focused way, to elicit hope, aspirations, strengths and goals.

Chapter 8: The legal and ethical landscape
(Charlotte Chisnell and Gordon Mitchell)

By discussing the recent changes that have been made in relation to mental health legislation, Charlotte and Gordon demonstrate how these changes are compatible with recent Government policy drivers that endorse a recovery model of service provision and enablement. This shows that the recent legislative changes set out to improve outcomes for people with mental health issues. However, they remind us that despite current policy promoting recovery and the involvement of the person with the mental health problem, ultimately the purpose of the majority of mental health legislations continues to focus on risk and protection.

Chapter 9: Enabling risk to aid recovery
(Angela Hall)

This chapter focuses not so much on Risk *within* recovery or the risks inherent in engaging in the Recovery Process, rather it explores the importance of risk and assessing and managing this to enable effective and safe recovery to take place. Angela explores the concept of risk and positive risk management in the context of contemporary mental health care planning. A recovery approach will be described when trying to measure and predict risk, and the need for a collaborative process in order to enable risks to be taken with the aim of promoting the person's journey of recovery. The chapter concludes with a case scenario that requires readers to consider decision making and risk taking in relation to promoting recovery as part of the care planning/planning care process.

Chapter 10: Collaborating across the boundaries
(Mike Wren, Stephan D. Kirby and Angela Hall)

By exploring the core features which are vital to any professional involved in the life of a person with mental health problems, the editors of this book demonstrate the necessity for effective collaboration. This is not only with the person with mental health problems but also from within an interprofessional working context. This chapter also demonstrates the importance for each professional to explore and understand the influences, philosophies and approaches that enhance and sustain such collaborations. By doing so, we can only benefit and enhance our practice and our work with people with mental health problems. This is a challenge to the traditional silo thinking that (unfortunately) still exists.

Chapter 11: Relationships and recovery
(Stephan D. Kirby)

The power behind successful recovery is the relationship between the person with the mental health problem and the mental health professional. In this chapter, Steve demonstrates how the traditional, paternalistic relationship is both damaging and infantilising, and the way forward, for the sake of the person with mental health problems, is the development of a collaborative dynamic therapeutic alliance. Within this chapter, he discusses a Model of Therapeutic Alliances created following trans-European research that underpins the creation of such a dynamic partnership as they travel the road to recovery. It focuses on the fact that health care is a human activity and as such it is one where both parties grow and learn. The therapeutic alliance offers hope, the opportunity to grow and develop and, through its flexible power agenda, a mutual learning environment.

Chapter 12: Holistic care planning for recovery
(Devon Marston and Jenny Weinstein)

Devon and Jenny discuss how person-centred care planning must involve people with mental health problems and their families in all aspects of care planning. They clearly demonstrate, and advocate, that at every stage care planning must address all aspects of a person's life, not simply their medical condition. The adoption of a Recovery Approach to underpin planning care is essential. It is again through the use of the powerful vehicle of the personal narrative that the contributors demonstrate what is both bad and good with current mental health services and the way they are organised and delivered from the viewpoint of the people that matter most – the recipients of this service. A range of strategies are offered to ensure that recovery is fundamental to planning care.

Chapter 13: Recovery-orientated practice in education
(Mike Fleet)

Mike clearly shows how contemporary nurse education does not encourage, nor indeed prepare, the student mental health nurse to embrace the core values of recovery of self-determination and self-management, and hope and expectations. He demonstrates that there is a clear need for this to be rectified. By reminding us that recovery is not about cure, rather it is about reclaiming a satisfying and meaningful life, he proposes that we need to educate students to be able to develop hope-inspiring relationships. He shows how mental health nurse training curricula can, and should, move towards a clear and distinct recovery focus. The student mental health nurse should be taught how to use themselves and develop personal qualities that aid the recovery process of a person with mental health problems. There should also be a greater use of the person with mental health problems as a partner in this education, in everything from planning and delivering curriculum to mentoring and assessing students. He leaves us with the frank message that mental health nursing students do not enter the profession to be agents of social control, yet that is the way they are perceived and what they ultimately end up becoming and that it is time to challenge mental health nurse education to remove the 'us' and 'them' and actively promote the 'we'.

Chapter 14: The recovery journey
(Stephan D. Kirby)

In this 'mini' chapter, Steve illustrates how the editors captured the major themes and concepts that influenced and underpinned this text. A visual, and annotated, representation (The Recovery Journey) of these is offered to the reader as a way to understand the recovery process (as we see it). In this, our variant, the recovery journey, has three major domains (which also form the frame for this book): 'Survive', 'Manage' and 'Thrive'. This then describes the various phases of the recovery process and descriptions of the experiences that the person with mental health problems could (or does) encounter at each phase are offered. It shows the journey from mental health crisis to mental health recovery, one which we hope will be beneficial to, and aid the reader in their endeavours, be they practitioner, academic or a person with mental health problems or their carer.

Chapter 15: Conclusions: reflection on the future
(Stephan D. Kirby, Mike Wren and Angela Hall)

And…the conclusions draws together the major issues and themes of the text and leaves the reader (hopefully) with food for thought in their own Recovery practices.

Now we have introduced the individual chapters we would like, for one last time, to reacquaint you to the questions from the end of our last edition and at the start of this one. We kindly ask that, as you engage with this book (in whichever way suits you best, either submerging yourself or dipping your toes), you bear these in mind and then you can decide whether, or not, we have answered them effectively.

> *How different would services look if their primary focus was to enable people to use and develop their skills, make the most of their assets, and pursue their aspirations?;*

> *Would this not change, for the better, the experience of using services, and the relationship between workers, and those whom we serve?* (Repper & Perkins, 2003:11).

References

Anthony, W.A. (1993) Recovery from mental illness: the guiding vision of the mental health service system in the 1990's. *Psychosocial Rehabilitation Journal*, **16**, 11–23.

Appleby, L. (2007) *Breaking Down Barriers: The Clinical Case for Change*. Department of Health, London.

Australian Government (2003) *Australian Health Ministers National Mental Health Plan, 2003–2008*. Australian Government, Canberra (www.mentalhealth.gov.au).

Barker, P.J. (2001) The Tidal Model: developing an empowering, person centred approach to recovery within psychiatric and mental health nursing. *Journal of Psychiatric and Mental Health Nursing*, **8**, 233–240.

Barnes, M. & Bowl, R. (2001) *Taking Over the Asylum: Empowerment and Mental Health*. Palgrave, Basingstoke.

Coleman, R. (1999) *Recovery: An Alien Concept*. Handsell, Gloucester.

Davidson, L. (2008) *Recovery: Concepts and Application*. Devon Recovery Group. Sainsbury Centre for Mental Health, London (www.scmh.org.uk).

Department of Health (DoH) (1983) *The Mental Health Act 1983*. Department of Health, London.

Department of Health (2001) *The Expert Patient*. Department of Health, London.

Department of Health (2006) *Our Health, Our Care, Our Say*. Department of Health, London (www.dh.gov.uk/en/index.htm).

Department of Health (2007) *Commissioning Framework for Health and Well-being*. Department of Health, London (www.dh.gov.uk/en/index.htm).

Department of Health and Human Services (2003) *Achieving the Promise: Transforming Mental Health Care in America*. President's New Freedom Commission on Mental Health, Pub no. SMA-03-3832. Department of Health and Human Services, Rockville.

Hafford-Letchfield, T. (2009) *Management and Organisations in Social Work*, Transforming Social Work Practice Series, 2nd edn. Learning Matters, Exeter.

Kaplan, G. (1964) *Principles of Preventative Psychiatry*. Tavistock, London.

Kirby, S.D. (2001) The development of a conceptual framework of therapeutic alliance in psychiatric (nursing) care delivery. In: *Forensic Mental Health: Working with the Mentally Ill Offender* (eds G. Landsberg & A. Smiley). pp. 25:1–25:8. Civic Research Institute, Kingston.

Kirby, S.D. & Cross, D.J. (2002) Socially constructed narrative intervention: a foundation for therapeutic alliances. In: *Therapeutic Interventions for Forensic Mental Health Nurses* (eds A. Kettles, P. Woods & M. Collins). pp. 187–205. Jessica Kingsley Publishers, London.

Larsen, J.A. (2004) Finding meaning in first episode psychosis: experience, agency and the cultural repertoire. *Medical Anthropology Quarterly*, **18**, 447–471.

Mental Health Commission (1998) *Blueprint for Mental Health Services in New Zealand*. Mental Health Commission, Wellington.

Mental Health Commission (2005) *A Vision for a Recovery Model in Irish Mental Health Services*. Mental Health Commission, Dublin.

Repper, J. & Perkins, R. (2003) *Social Inclusion and Recovery: A Model for Mental Health Practice*. Elsevier Health Sciences, Edinburgh.

Rogers, A. & Pilgrim, D. (2010) *A Sociology of Mental Health and Illness*, 4th edn. McGraw-Hill Education, Maidenhead.

Romme, M. & Escher, S. (1993) *Accepting Voices*. MIND Publications, London.

Saleebey, D. (2009) *The Strengths Perspective in Social Work Practice*, 4th edn. Allyn & Bacon, Boston.

Scotland Government (2006) *Rights, Relationships and Recovery: The Report of the National Review of Mental Health Nursing in Scotland* [Online]. Available at www. scotland.gov.uk/Publications/2006/04/18164814/0. Accessed on April 30, 2013.

Shepherd, G., Boardman, J. & Slade, M. (2008) *Making Recovery a Reality*. Sainsbury Centre for Mental Health, London.

Watkins, P. (2001) *Mental Health Nursing: The Art of Compassionate Care*. Butterworth-Heinemann, London.

White, M. & Epston, D. (1990) *Narrative Means to Therapeutic Ends*. Norton, New York.

Chapter 2

Experiencing Recovery

Aidan Moesby and Sandra Cleminson

Teesside University, UK

If you have 100 people in a room with a diagnosis of a specific mental health condition, you will have 100 different symptoms and behaviours. Everybody experiences their 'condition' uniquely. Similarly, everybody experiences recovery uniquely. However, there are well-documented commonalities that contribute to the process.

Recovery is not a one-way journey; there will be set backs of varying orders. We all know life is not static, we are on *the* continuum of good days and bad days, mentally well and mentally unwell. Our needs change and how we cope changes. Continually self-monitoring, attempting to stay at the top of our game, is not only exhausting but tiresome. Watching for triggers, checking how busy we are, how we are coping, whether we are getting enough sleep or eating properly all whilst trying to live our life at the same time. I want to live the most enriched and fulfilled life possible, and I do not want to be self-monitoring and adapting continually. Therein lies the conflict, and I am forever walking the tightrope of degrees of latitude. Too much monitoring and I limit the mindfulness of being in the moment, too little and I risk falling into the chaos I am attempting to circumvent.

Experiencing any acute/severe mental health condition can be very isolating. It can be very life limiting and reduce opportunities to lead a varied and fulfilled life. Diagnosis can often be preceded by a crisis, which can be scary for those around us to witness. This can lead to a rapid shrinking in our social and professional worlds. Even after diagnosis where stabilisation may have occurred, life can still be very chaotic.

Recovery is enhanced by doing activities that make us feel better about ourselves, which affirm our place in the world. Recovery is not a one-way journey. Indeed, recognising there will be set-backs, of varying orders, is important. The temptation to self-punish and vilify for the perceived failure must be

Care Planning in Mental Health: Promoting Recovery, Second Edition.
Edited by Angela Hall, Michael Wren and Stephan D. Kirby.
© 2013 John Wiley & Sons, Ltd. Published 2013 by John Wiley & Sons, Ltd.

resisted; for it may deepen the setback and prolong the next steps to recovery. Accepting that this is all part of the process can be used as a reflective learning experience. Understanding that we need to be gentle on ourselves can contribute to a much more positive and holistic view of 'Recovery'.

My recovery is a combination of understanding what makes me well, what makes me unwell, rejecting or avoiding versus embracing and encouraging. When I first got diagnosed, I did not have a clue about anything. My moods were highly erratic, my life was suddenly populated by professionals that came in pairs and I had been parachuted into that foreign country of the service user and psychiatrist – thankfully, I mastered the basics of the language quite quickly. Following the acute episode of mental ill health that preceded my diagnosis, I lost my job, house, relationship and experienced the abandonment of friends. Had it not been for the support I received from my sister and remaining close friends at this crucial time, my life could have been very different. Without this vital safety net, I would probably have ended up on the streets, with all the consequences that this entails. The support and guidance to make the sometimes difficult decisions, the assistance with the practical things needed to facilitate the necessary changes and the ensuring I was getting the professional services I needed were significant factors in arresting my decline. The first six weeks postdiagnosis were incredibly difficult, not just the day-to-day struggle of managing even primary functions but the coming to terms with what living with a diagnosis of Bipolar Affective Disorder means.

I was fortunate to be rehoused in a great flat in a very liveable town and fall under the care of a fantastic Psychiatrist and supported by an understanding CPN. I did not know it then, but I was already constructing my own recovery. Regular clinical appointments saw my medication rise on a steep upward curve. My moods may have stabilised, but I had stopped being aware of the world. I was looking out through the thousand yard stare. I had slipped into an anaesthetised existence, going through the motions of living. I was unable to work and barely socialised. My life had become incredibly limited.

My Psychiatrist would ask me what makes me feel better about things as I complained of low self-esteem, low confidence and other deficits that affect my wellbeing. As an artist, making 'work' feeds me and allows me to feel positive about myself, doing 'work' for, and with, others benefits me through socialisation, whilst engaged in something I consider worthwhile. In order to make 'work', I need to be able to feel things and respond, to imagine and then create. Medication had taken this away from me. Then my Psychiatrist said 'What do you want to do about it'? That was a pivotal point in my recovery. There I was being asked what I wanted, and I had a real say in my own care; I was in a dialogue. Then the coup-de-gras, 'You are the expert in your own condition'. I couldn't believe what I was hearing. The feeling of autonomy was palpable.

I reduced my medication, my drug induced haze and torpor subsided. I began to feel connected to the world again, albeit in a small way at first. I began to experience the world in a much more proactive and engaged manner. The world took on a vividness and crispness, my sense of separation and alienation faded, and I was no longer a passive spectator in my own life. This reawakening enabled me to make 'work' and create, and I was ready and more able to socialise and be among people. I was slowly able to fill the acute sense of emptiness I had felt inside. My confidence increased, I felt better about myself and I liked myself more – I was participating in my own life and it felt good again.

I began to expand my world. I could get back on the train and goto the city, arrange to meet someone in a cafe or go to the movies; everyday activities for most people. In the early days of recovery, these were extraordinary achievements for me. My CPN was also instrumental in turning things around. He had a wholly collaborative approach. I tended to use him as a sounding board, to reflect on things that had happened and to look at alternative strategies that I could implement when in difficulty – both emotionally and physically. He would lead when I said I was stuck, given choices I could choose a solution that felt right for me at the time. Of course when I am not so well, I slip into my old patterns – but I can live with that. Small victories are important and small backward steps are not the end of the world.

Much of my recovery has been about creating a safety matrix. I have three general phases, Surviving; Managing and Thriving. When I am surviving, I go back to what I know best and that which keeps me safest. Familiar roads taken, sit in the same seat that kind of thing. When I am thriving, I can expand my world, try new things, and this increases my options of things being safe when I am just surviving. It is not just about being reactive, finding myself in a situation and then trying to cope with it. Much of my recovering is about creativity and expansion – as if I were an athlete in training for the next event – constantly.

When I had reduced my medication significantly and was consistently stable, I returned to work – experiencing all those associated benefits of increases in wellbeing, confidence and esteem. At this time, I met a lecturer who introduced me to the notion of 'User Engagement'. I liked the reasoning and theories behind it, and my curiosity was such that I agreed to take part in one of the sessions. However, I baulk at the terminology around 'User Engagement' or 'User Involvement' in the same way that I really do not like the stigmatising labels and language around mental health I find them disempowering, demeaning, deskilling and dehumanising. My identity as an individual is subsumed by various systems and professional bodies. This has a major impact on how I feel about myself. Yes I do have a diagnosis, but I still want to be seen as an individual with individual characteristics, qualities and skills.

User engagement at its worst is wheeling in people like circus freaks to be stared at, tell their story and be metaphorically poked and prodded.

Thankfully, my experience was altogether more positive. I want to make a difference to those who come behind me. I want to challenge the inequalities and the stigma, not just among the general public but the professional services too. I was initially asked to present a narrative at an interprofessional learning day, an attempt at joined-up thinking between varying professionals involved in complex cases. It was a positive experience; I felt valued, listened to and respected and that what I was contributing was being taken seriously. I began sharing my story with students at University on Health and Social Care courses.

At the same time, I began to get involved with my local User Networks. One thing had led to another. One experience was leverage for the next. This has developed into more active involvement in devising and delivering sessions with the same lecturer for more than four years. This has been a fantastic opportunity and one which is largely collaborative in the true sense of the word – obviously she has ultimate responsibility but we discuss what works, what has not, what would be good to include and how we could develop the working relationship. It has developed into a long-term collaborative relationship, which has included lecturing, writing a paper and presenting at conference. I am encouraged to lead but I know the support is there if I stumble. The power dynamics are delicate. I know I have a degree of autonomy – this is freely given. This is a core collaborative community for me. It has a reach far wider though. The experience, the leverage, the impact on what it means to me all keep me moving forward, recovering through supported challenges. Initially, I thought my involvement in user engagement was altruistic but it was later I realised it was more than this. In fact, it was one of the key moments in recognising things about myself and my own recovery. I now train, lecture and mentor around the subject and the wider field of disability and equality.

I have invested a lot in building a sustainable community around me. It has taken 7 years to reach the stage I am at now, and it is still a work in progress. There is no room for smugness. Relapses are a great leveller and a good time to reflect on things.

As much as I have actively sought to create and engage in collaborative supportive relationships, the medical ones have been just as important. This is a tale of two towns though. I had seen psychiatry from a professional capacity, and such was my horror I resisted getting assessed until I could no longer deny my need or manage my increasingly severe episodes. My Psychiatrist for the first 6 years of diagnosis changed my opinion of the psychiatric services. Even though I knew very little at the start, when I was asked how I was, I would then be asked how I thought things could be improved and then what did I think would improve them. So, for example, I knew things had slightly improved because of my medication; therefore, I was willing and compliant to go with a negotiated increase in drugs. My Psychiatrist would not just deal with the medical or the psychological;

my appointments always included aspects of exploring the psycho-social and the personal. He understood how one impacts on another.

I felt very much an equal in this relationship. I knew ultimately where the power lay, but he strived to share it as much as possible. Nothing was done without my consultation or approval. When I was describing how I was feeling after a reduction in medication, he would say: 'Well, we can up it, down it, or just keep it the same – what do you think?' This is incredibly empowering. It gives a sense that you are at the forefront of your own recovery, creating a model for yourself, albeit a guided one. Having things explained and information shared adds to this, it enables me to make informed decisions – so knowing that reducing my mood stabilisers might precipitate a manic swing, and therefore I may have to take something to counter this is empowering. This regime change is not just something that happens to me, and I am very much part of the process. But that is my point, in the same way as I wanted supported challenges in the User Expert endeavours, similarly I needed the support and guidance of my psychiatrist. In addition, knowing that if we did change the regime that I could access services if need be. There was a joined-up system.

My doctors, in a rural practice, had a CPN in surgery. The doctors fostered fantastic relationships. I rarely used the extra services available to me but when required I could book after surgery sessions for extended periods that would act as a maintenance or holding service until I was back into the secondary services proper. Then I could access the CPN without waiting for weeks on end for a referral. I was segued back into the support I needed. This relationship was developed over several years; it was individual to me. We constructed it together from learning what works and what does not, what keeps me well and what contributes to a decline in my mental wellbeing. Largely, it kept me well and functioning at a high level. I could work and maintain my relationships; I was mostly within my managing and thriving scale rather than just surviving.

The other advantage to this is twofold. I do not have a dependence on services created or fostered, and second, and perhaps more importantly, I am kept from acute decline. I know the further I go down in mood and functioning and the longer it lasts, the harder it is and longer it takes to recover. The whole model was about maintenance and recovery. It was focused around negotiated practice, shared responsibility and collaboration.

Counter to this is the care I received when I moved to a different district. There was no joined-up approach, no seamless moving between services and indeed, seemingly, a complete lack of services. Twice I referred myself for assessment and twice I was refused any secondary care. I had no Care Manager, CPN, psychiatrist or any another form of support. Needless to say, my mental health declined consistently and acutely.

Recovery is not a one-way journey. By its very nature it has setbacks, stumbles, falls within it. Recovery is cyclical. The key is to build up enough resilience in order to overcome these setbacks so they do not completely disarm us and we find ourselves acutely unwell. Through building a flexible/ supple psychology where we can respond more appropriately to challenges, we can take ourselves further into recovery with each little advancement and development. Recovery is not a journey made in isolation. I cannot do it alone. Despite having a high degree of insight and awareness into my own condition and pathology, I do need support from professionals, friends and family. The aforementioned collaborative relationships are vital for this. The tendency to discharge early and take away support has had a detrimental effect upon my own recovery. It is quite simple – what happens when the CPN, Psychologist, Psychiatrist or Care Coordinator are taken away is that it leaves me feeling totally uncontained. Whilst these professionals remain in place, I may in fact never access them, just knowing they are available is enough to 'hold me'. Should the case arise when I do need them they are readily accessible without having to go through the time-consuming process of attempting to get back 'in the system' through assessment teams. The time saved by accessing services has a beneficial impact on my mental health as I do not get so unwell. It is clear that the more acutely unwell people get, the time to move back into meaningful recovery is extended.

The longer I am in recovery, the more resilience and inner strength I develop, thus making relapse less likely, or should I say the things that would trigger a relapse tend to be the more significant (and generally less frequent) events. Moving out of recovery, relapsing into acute unwellness or episodes of disorder is not just about being unwell. This can be seen and felt as a failure, which can lead to self-punishment for not continually succeeding, not meeting or living up to my own, unrealistically high, expectations of myself. This can, and tends to, exacerbate the spiral of decent into unwellness. The associated feelings of failure maybe prevalent and lead to a return to low esteem, low self-confidence and associated factors. Of course, the converse is true – maintaining the positive collaborative relationships can assist in the maintenance of the recovery journey. At the outset, I may have one particular view of how recovery, my recovery, may look to me. However, this view is dynamic, it is not set in stone and THAT is my recovery mapped and modelled forever. My initial opinion of what I need may change. How I expand my world, the opportunities that present, the choices that I make , how aware I remain – there are always hidden obstacles that may trip me up. Recovery is an evolutionary, if not revolutionary journey.

Current literature offers clear messages from service users in terms of the types of services they have identified as being most useful to support recovery in mental health. This should mean, services are able to provide what users want. It sounds simple, but in reality, it appears that some areas do provide this and others do not. There are clear indicators of what service users need and how they want this to be delivered. It seems the direction forward is clear but obscured. In an attempt to side step this, Aidan and myself have agreed that his story should focus on what went well in his experience. His narrative highlights how services can meet the needs of those who need them and it includes issues to consider for those of us who care about what happens next. In order for mental health services to support recovery, they should be tailor-made to the individual and led by those who use them. The development and delivery of future services should be less reliant on government changes and be directed by those who use them. They should be available in the shape and form of what is required on a spectrum of support that is accessible, prevents relapse, empowers and is flexible to need, whilst fostering independence and self-reliance.

Recommended reading

Blank, A. & Hayward, M. (2009) The role of work in recovery. *British Journal of Occupational Therapy*, **72** (7), 324–326.

Clouston, T. (2003) Narrative methods: talk, listening and representation. *British Journal of Occupational Therapy*, **66** (4), 136–142.

College of Occupational Therapists (2006) *Recovering Ordinary Lives, The Strategy for Occupational Therapy Services 2007–2017*. College of Occupational Therapists, London.

Fieldhouse, J. (2012) Community participation and recovery for mental health service users: an action research inquiry. *British Journal of Occupational Therapy*, **75** (9), 419–428.

Smyth, G., Harries, P. & Dorer, G. (2011) Exploring mental health service users' experiences of social inclusion in their community occupations. *British Journal of Occupational Therapy*, **74** (7), 323–331.

Chapter 3

Recovery as a Framework for Care Planning

Jim Campbell,[1] *Theo Stickley,*[2] *Sarah Bonney*[3] *and Nicola Wright*[4]

[1] Self-employed Mental Health Trainer, UK
[2] University of Nottingham, UK
[3] British Columbia Children's Hospital, Canada
[4] Collaboration for Leadership in Applied Health Research and Care (CLAHRC), UK

> *What matters is not whether we're using services or not using services; using medications or not using medications. What matters in terms of a recovery orientation is, are we living the life we want to be living? Are we achieving the life we want to be living? Are we achieving personal goals? Do we have friends? Do we have connections with the community? Are we contributing or giving back in some way?* (Deegan, 1993)

Introduction

Pat Deegan's statement captures the essence of recovery; of how anyone who has experienced mental distress could be living. In this chapter, we discuss how the mental health practitioner might provide an environment where the individual is supported and facilitated in achieving a life that is meaningful for them. With the growing concept of recovery within mental health services, there needs to be a change in the way mental health professionals work in the future with people who have experienced mental distress. We aim to provide mental health practitioners with a broad understanding of the many issues around successfully developing recovery-focused work and we aim to provide ideas for developing frameworks needed for care planning that promote the true essence of recovery.

Care Planning in Mental Health: Promoting Recovery, Second Edition.
Edited by Angela Hall, Michael Wren and Stephan D. Kirby.
© 2013 John Wiley & Sons, Ltd. Published 2013 by John Wiley & Sons, Ltd.

We approach this whole subject with temerity. As authors, we have all been trained as mental health professionals. Although we may acknowledge our own mental distress, none of us has been hospitalised under the Mental Health Act (DoH, 1983) or been diagnosed with an enduring mental health problem. While some authors on recovery have their feet in both camps, we do not. We recognise from the outset therefore that we are not the most qualified people to write about this subject. As professionals though, we are able to appreciate the service-user discourse on recovery and act as translators, interpreters or advocates to the world of mental health practice. What we are blatantly aware of is the potential for the concept of recovery to be hijacked by the professional discourse. In 2009, the Sainsbury Centre (now known as the Centre for Mental Health) presented a framework for organisational change which consisted of ten key challenges that need to be addressed by mental health services if they are to become more recovery orientated. It could be argued that what is understood by some as a service-user movement is all too quickly becoming a statutory vehicle for service delivery. Further embedding recovery within the professional lexicon are posts such as 'Fellows for Recovery' at Universities and the increasing number of courses focusing on recovery for a professional audience (e.g., the MA in Recovery and Social Inclusion at the University of Nottingham). What began its life as a movement or paradigm is fast becoming a method for systems. We do not wish to contribute to that process; rather, we wish to encourage mental health workers to appreciate the depth of meaning of the concept of recovery and apply this meaning to their work. Furthermore, the notion of recovery carries with it a set of values that puts the position of the service user as paramount within the hierarchy of care. If our book-chapter contributes to this in some small way, then we will have achieved much.

What is becoming increasingly acknowledged is that although the ideas and values of recovery are becoming embraced and taken on board, it is a lot less clear how to embed these into practice. This has taken the recovery movement into a new era within the UK with the formation of new organisations to enable recovery practices.

The chapter will consider the concept of recovery with its values and principles, providing the reader with a foundation upon which they might be able to practice mental health care in a more meaningful way. This is largely achieved through a review of the recovery literature, paying particular attention to what writers have been saying in recent years. We consider recovery in the light of social construct theory and discuss the implications of this understanding for mental health practice. We draw on service-user experiences and some of their concerns and fears. Examples of recovery philosophies, models and approaches will then be addressed, providing questions on whether working within the particular frameworks captures the essence of recovery. Finally, the chapter considers some alternative approaches, drawing on examples for the reader to consider. It is hoped that the reader will begin to understand some of the complexities and issues around developing a recovery framework, enabling them to reflect on their own practices within the future.

Recovery debated

Recovery is being increasingly debated within mental health discourse. It appears to have a multitude of meanings, such as an idea, a movement, a philosophy, a set of values, policy and a doctrine for change (Turner, 2002a). It has split opinion: on the one hand, it is viewed as simplistic, and on the other, revolutionary. Various models of recovery are being postulated: the National Institute for Mental Health in England (NIMHE, 2004); Barker (2001); Copeland (2006); Fisher (2005); Heather (2002); The National Institute for Clinical Excellence (NICE, 2002b); Repper & Perkins (2003); Rethink (2005); May *et al.* (1999) and more recently, CHIME (connectedness, hope and optimism about the future, identity, meaning in life and empowerment (Leamy *et al.*, 2011)). Within the UK (and elsewhere), recovery as a concept has been operationalised and used as a means to change organisational culture and to plan and deliver mental health services. Recovery teams have been operating for some years (DoH, 1999) and more recently, under the auspices of the Centre for Mental Health, the ImRoC (Implementing Recovery through Organisational Change) project has piloted a framework for organisation change to assist service provision to become more recovery orientated. Embracing the growing virtual work, Working to Recovery and International Mental Health Collaborating Network has formed ICRA-Whole Life (The International Centre for Recovery Action in Practice Education and Research) creating a nongeographically based centre to embed recovery practices into all aspects of life (see http://www.icra-wholelife.org/).

Recovery has therefore a growing impetus within the UK. In other parts of the world, for example, New Zealand, Australia and North America, recovery as a concept in mental health services has become well established. Despite the growth of recovery within the UK and elsewhere, the literature surrounding the concept indicates that there still needs to be changes in the way mental health professionals work if the ethos of recovery is to be maintained. The traditional role of providing individual services, based on what the professional thinks to be most appropriate, will need to be replaced with a comprehensive system to support the service users to achieve their chosen goals:

Adopting a recovery approach in a community mental health system (as contrasted with simply incorporating language about recovery in policy documents) necessitates fundamental changes in the ways that needs are assessed, and how services are planned, delivered and evaluated (Grierson, 2001:4).

The voice of the service user will need to be at the centre of their own care; they will be seen as the expert on their experiences, deciding on the form of their care and support, whether it is social, medical, psychological and/or educational. The mental health professionals' role will shift from the traditional role of being the expert, to working alongside service users and carers as peers in supporting them to make these choices and decisions. This will give the service user hope and empowerment for their future, from their often poor experiences of the psychiatric system (Mead & Copeland, 2000; Coleman *et al.*, 2001):

> *There will need to be major organisational changes to challenge policies and proce-*
> *dures that prevent recovery practices. Recovery, not treatment, will need to be*
> *placed at the centre of all practices, enabling the formation of a service where prac-*
> *titioners work to support and facilitate service users in a recovery focused way*
> (Campbell & Gallagher, 2007:33).

What perhaps is most challenging for mental health workers is not the necessary change to systems and approaches, but rather the change that is required within one's self. Working in a recovery-orientated manner is intrinsically linked with personal beliefs and values.

The key to the recovery concept is the simple premise that recovery from enduring mental health problems is possible. Historically, people who have been diagnosed with a mental illness have been told that their symptoms are incurable and that they will have to take medication for the rest of their lives; they will never work, get married or have children. With the growing literature from personal experiences of service users, professionals and research, over the last few decades, it has been clearly demonstrated that recovery is possible (Mead & Copeland, 2000; Deegan, 2001).

> *The consumer/survivor movement has shown that through empowerment and*
> *peer support even people with the most 'hopeless' diagnosis, schizophrenia, can*
> *recover fully* (Ahern & Fisher, 2001:24).

These are not merely theoretical postulations. Writers including Ron Coleman (2011) and Rufus May (2000a) have demonstrated from their own experiences that people who have been hospitalised, heavily medicated, felt despair and hopelessness for the future can recover. They have shown that people can confront their experiences and live meaningful functional lives within society.

Historical context

The idea of recovery in mental ill-health can be traced back more than 200 years and was instrumental in informing the philosophy of the Tukes at the York Retreat. It has been suggested that RD Laing and the antipsychiatric movement 'planted a seed' that helped propel people with schizophrenia towards recovery (Kelly & Gamble, 2005). Rethink (2005) cites Dr. Abraham Low as having developed the first recovery approach in 1930 when he set up post in-patient self-help groups to enhance self-determination and develop self-confidence. The physical disability movement and de-institutionalisation within psychiatry led to the emergence of a recovery vision in America in the 1990s. New Zealand has also followed this philosophy and in the United Kingdom recovery has followed on from disability legislation, antidiscrimination and consumerism and the civil rights movements of the 1960s and 1970s. The sharing of personal accounts has further developed this concept and helped to reduce stigma (Roberts & Wolfson, 2004).

The concept of recovery emerged from those people who had first-hand experience of mental health difficulties (Repper & Perkins, 2003) and is arguably a political response to an unsatisfactory mental health system that focuses on maintenance (Turner, 2002a). The National Schizophrenia Fellowship in Powys compiled a report on the recovery approach in 2001 (Turner & Frak, 2001). Their review identified three models of modern care:

- Medical: 'We can treat you/we can cure you'.
- Social: 'You have needs that we should meet'.
- Recovery: 'I have a problem that I can grow beyond with help'.

The purpose of the review was to explore the perspectives and meaning associated with the concept of recovery. The promotion of recovery was thought to involve the worker assuming a nonexpert role, with the service user as the expert of their own experience. This was a shift away from the medical paradigm. It was possible that issues of risk, responsibility, choice and policy-making were at odds with current systems. The question was therefore to explore whether service delivery was complementary to the experience of recovery for individuals. From this, the paper went on to identify conflicting and common views and demonstrate potential areas of service shortfall. While it may be useful to identify models of care to promote recovery (we develop this later), firstly, we need to understand more about how the concept of recovery is constructed.

The mental health literature regarding recovery could be divided into what may be referred to as 'discourses'. In other words, the meaning of the word 'recovery' is largely dependent on the perspective of the person who is defining it. People's perspectives are determined by their life experiences. Each of us 'constructs' our own versions of the world. In the case of recovery, understandably, the person with a diagnosis of mental health problems will have a very different perspective to the person who has given the diagnosis. Collectively, we could identify a 'service user discourse' and a 'service provider discourse'. However, the distinctions are not that straightforward as some people who provide services are also people who have used services. There is a branch of social science that deals with this concept that is called 'Social Constructionism'. Later in this chapter, we consider the concept of recovery from a social constructionist perspective. Before this, we will look at what the recovery literature actually tells us about recovery and mental health. Recent literature has been analysed and we present the themes from this analysis.

Recovery concepts in the literature

Recent literature reviews focusing on recovery in mental health indicate that as a concept it is extremely complex. As we have identified in the opening pages of this chapter, recovery in mental health incorporates multiple agendas including the political, organisational and social. It also emphasises themes such as hope, optimism, power and finding meaning in life. The evidence relating to recovery also incorporates many different voices (as we shall demonstrate later in this chapter, recovery can be said to be socially constructed) and unsurprisingly the type of literature which forms the evidence base is extremely diverse. For example, academic studies published in peer-reviewed journals and subjected to scientific rigour as well as service-user accounts of their own recovery and experiences of mental health services published in nonpeer reviewed or 'grey' sources. By highlighting the diversity of literature available relating to recovery in mental health, we do not wish to suggest that some offer more valid accounts of recovery in mental health than others. Indeed, given the risk of recovery becoming subsumed by professionals, the importance of maintaining and valuing the service-user voice within the evidence base is crucial.

Drawing on four reviews conducted since 2008 (Bonney & Stickley, 2008; Leamy *et al.*, 2011; Stickley & Wright, 2011a; Stickley & Wright, 2011b), we outline some of the broad themes emerging from the literature related to recovery in mental health. Although these themes will be presented separately and sequentially, they also interweave; that is, a particular study, article or book may fall into one or several of the themes. The six themes to be discussed are:

1) The intrapersonal domain;
2) The service provision agenda, including activities/interventions which promote recovery;
3) The social domain;
4) Power and control;
5) Hope and optimism;
6) Risk and responsibility.

The intrapersonal domain

Recovery, described interpersonally, is a theme dominated by service users and steeped in individual stories and closely tied to issues of identity. Recovery is often defined in terms of an on-going process requiring a change in attitudes and values (Repper & Perkins, 2003). It is also identified with learning and growth (Fisher, 2000; Turner, 2002b; Whitehill, 2003) and a conversion from coping to healing (Fisher, 2000; Repper & Perkins, 2003). Barker (2003) elaborates further by speculating that the healing may be discovered during the journey itself, rather than upon reaching any final destination. In essence, it is a highly personal journey which may be helped or hindered by the actions of others (Whitehall, 2009). 'Others' in this context could include mental health professionals, and flexible services are considered essential in order to provide individually tailored care. However, Repper & Ford (2006) identifies that often service user and professional views may compete or conflict. Furthermore, societal level approaches can fail to account for local and personal needs (DoH, 2003). For example, the Mental Health Foundation (2004) states that public attitudes towards mental health (which often have a strong influence on policy developments) can impose limits on an individual's potential to achieve recovery.

Within this context, a person's experience is considered fluid (Barker, 2000) and as uniquely individual journey (Fisher, 2000; Turner & Frak, 2001; MacDonald, 2005). Indeed, for some people, mental illness may not be a wholly negative experience and can potentially enrich and add meaning to an individual's life. Roberts *et al.* (2008) suggests that mental distress can add meaning to one's life as the experience increases self-awareness and personal growth. The significance of recovery for Deegan (1993) was not to attain 'normality' but to embark on the recovery journey to realise one's calling. Recovery here does not stand still, but is an ongoing process of personal discovery (Turner, 2002a; Wimberley & Peters, 2003; Kelly & Gamble, 2005).

The personal aspect of individual recovery defined, lived and managed by service users, whilst highlighted within policy rhetoric, can become filtered and diluted as the practicalities of service provision are meted out, focusing on outcomes (DoH, 1999; Reid *et al.*, 2001; Blair, 2004). The language can become paternalistic, with providers seeking to stabilise people's conditions (Lester *et al.*, 2005), with preferred service-user behaviour being modelled from universal and generic practice (NIMHE, 2004). The development of such models, whilst enabling service providers and policy-makers with measurable evidence and statistics, may inadvertently stifle the individuality and creativity they are seeking to promote (Turner & Frak, 2001), unless measurement of success remains firmly within the service-user domain (Holloway, 2002).

Service provision agenda

Despite there being a general consensus around placing service-user needs first (DoH 1999; Sainsbury Centre for Mental Health, 2001; DoH, 2001, 2002; NICE, 2002a; NIMHE, 2003, 2004, 2005; DoH, 2005; WHO, 2005), one might question whose best interests are served by maintaining a model that promotes the 'ill-cured' dichotomy. To attempt to eradicate and at best 'manage' an individual's experiences not only retains a strong 'marriage' to the pharmaceutical industry but also influences society and community in terms of acceptability and what is permitted.

Groups that describe recovery in terms of a biomedical model, seek an absence of symptoms. Campbell (2001) describes providers wanting to eliminate problems as opposed to expose or integrate them. Crucially, recovery is considered to be achievable without cure. The Sainsbury Centre for Mental Health (2001) declares that 'mental health services aim to cure or ameliorate ill health' (p. 3). The National Institute for Mental Health in England (NIMHE) website provides information booklets in association with a pharmaceutical company. Chalmers (2001) argues that the pharmaceutical industry has 'hijacked' mental health care with biomedical frameworks increasing their domination in education and research. Some observers argue that hidden promotion can be located in research funding, with pharmaceutical companies infiltrating hospitals and universities who are short of public funding, by providing contract-based research, often not open to public scrutiny (Mansfield & Jureidini, 2001).

If recovery is referred to in terms of 'complete cure' or getting back to 'normal', then few people will recover (Roberts & Wolfson, 2004). The DoH & Hope (2004) state that 'recovery is not about eliminating symptoms or the notion of cure', and Harrison *et al.* (2001) define complete recovery as 'no longer requiring any treatment'. Policy, however, tends to focus on these very issues (Roberts & Wolfson, 2004). NICE & National Collaborating Centre for Mental Health (2003) state that medication is viewed as indispensable for most people in a recovery phase and Travis *et al.* (2001) record its efficacious role in prevention. Buckingham (2001) and May (2001) argue that medication only serves to suppress symptoms and hinder recovery as a result of dissociation unless one can confront the unconscious world in order to make sense of what has happened.

Coleman (2011) argues that recovery occurs within the context of complex relationships. It involves every aspect of the human condition, thus is truly holistic (Turner, 2002a). Coleman (2011) states that the mental health system can destroy the fragile sense of self by explaining experiences and problems as biological, labelling attempts to find a voice as lack of insight and seeing anger and fear as aggression and deterioration. Thus, the essential components of recovery that Coleman outlines as the four 'selfs' are, he believes, undermined by the very system set up to help. He notes that this often subsides into a loss of identity and eventual compliance, leading to denial of the experience.

Warner (2004) argues that 114 follow-up studies of outcome in schizophrenia (conducted in the developed world since the beginning of the twentieth century) showed recovery rates were no better for those admitted post the introduction of antipsychotic medication than for those predating this period. Despite this, a model of deficits and pathology has been in the ascension for many years, with a present emphasis on maintenance and relapse prevention (May, 2000b).

The emphasis on the 'medical' management of mental distress can also restrict mental health services and professionals from exploring other (nonmedical) activities which could promote recovery. Involvement in arts initiatives, education, employment and physical activity have all been found to be beneficial to individuals and enhance recovery. For example, through developing coping strategies, increasing self-expression, improved social support networks and rebuilding identity (Spandler *et al.*, 2007; Carless & Douglas, 2008).

There is great diversity of feeling around the philosophy of recovery even amongst those who use services, with recovery and the medical model exhibiting significant tensions (Roberts & Wolfson, 2004). Jacobson (2004) argues that these tensions can be alleviated by accepting the individuality and uniqueness of recovery, but goes on to state that this approach presents difficulties for policy makers. There are, however, numerous authors within the literature who advocate recovery in its wider terms, and Nolan (2000) states that recent scholarship points to a 'middle way' that recognises the value of both. Recovery appears hotly contested within the service provision arena with money, power and control underpinning decision-making. Groups may have an invested interest in maintaining the status quo, thus challenging attempts to seek a middle way.

The social domain

Coleman (2011) asserts that one cannot become whole if isolated from society. Furthermore, Barker and Buchanan-Barker (2003) argue that recovery can and does take place in the absence of treatment and can occur with the right kind of social support. Here, recovery is seen as being dependent on a variety of other external factors, such as the environment, civil rights and opportunities for inclusion (Sayce, 2000). Indeed, as Warner (2004) identifies, the recovery movement may have its roots in asylum closure but the contemporary literature which supports recovery also endorses the theme of promoting social inclusion. However, Coleman (2011) questions the reality of social recovery, arguing that the mental health system in effect robs people of opportunities to develop social and economic independence through stigmatisation and institutionalisation. Campbell (2001) describes his experience: 'Ever since I was catapulted from the status of under-graduate scholar to that of long term mental patient questions about who I am now have been central' (p. 16). This is further explored by the British Psychological Society (2000) which talks of the need to recover from prejudice, stigma, low expectations and the pressure to adhere to a 'sick role'. Similarly, although the desire for social inclusion may be considered one of social justice (Repper & Perkins, 2009), the political emphasis upon people accessing employment and the personalisation agenda (DoH, 2009) has meant that social inclusion has also become synonymous with getting people off social security benefits and cost-cutting.

Furthermore, there may be powerful social forces at work that may militate against recovery. For example, there may be incongruity between the rhetoric of policy-makers and the actual lived experience of service users, where accessing meaningful work, living in an environment conducive to health, overcoming prejudice and being genuinely included in the formation of services are often not the norms (Martyn, 2002).

Deegan's (2001) personal experience was of others 'seeing' schizophrenia before they saw her or her potential to work. Furthermore, she outlined the importance of living in an environment tolerant of difference. Even if policy and service provision promote social inclusion, resistance may occur within communities. Additionally, if full integration is realised for some, stigma may prevent the true attainment of potential and lost career years may never be recouped unless education, careers and financial support can be tailored to individual's needs and discrimination abolished. Stanton (2001) found an application to enter Australia failed due to the applicant being sectioned under the Mental Health Act in the past. It could therefore be argued that beyond the rhetoric of social inclusion and the value of homes, work and careers (ordinary things many take for granted), a number of obstacles stand in the way and serve to 'filter out' opportunities for recovering a social life. The whole business of recovery therefore cannot be separated from people's social issues including their social problems. Mental health problems are intertwined with social problems such as poverty, poor housing, racism, abuse, relationship breakdown and possible subsequent issues such substance misuse and dependency.

Power and control

The study of the literature illuminated underlying shifts of power, ownership and control around the emergence of recovery in contemporary health care. Coleman (2011) sees service users as a commodity that agencies 'bid' for, vying to provide services and obtain funding. He says that it will be essential for service users to reclaim power as a vital part of the recovery process. This view is mirrored by Barchard (2005) who argues that self-management is very often commandeered by the establishment.

Kendell (2000), speaking at a Royal College of Psychiatrists' annual meeting, expresses concerns over psychiatrists' perceived loss of power to other professions and service users'. He considers that the way of retaining power is through the continued management of medication and fears the loss of the sole right to prescribe. Power is also retained through the promotion of the medical model with Kendell seeing no fundamental difference between physical and mental illness. Furthermore, he offers a prediction that psychiatry will become more 'biological' in future and begin to catch up with other physical illnesses in terms of biochemical knowledge. The motivation behind the desire to listen to service users is not necessarily philanthropic as Kendell (2000) states that to refuse to listen or 'fall out' with service-user organisations could damage psychiatrists' reputations badly. Finances are also cited as being a driving force behind the choice and delivery of services, with the suspicion that funds will follow psychological services seen to be 'taken over' by clinical psychologists. Kendell expresses further concerns about a rise in consumerism, which he believes equates to a reduced deference towards the medical profession.

The control of symptoms often remains in the provider/policy-maker domains. The 12-year follow-up study of those regarded as 'heavy users' of psychiatric services by Reid *et al.* (2001) focused on assessing problems, deficits and needs. The authors concluded that to improve 'outcomes' for this 'group', further active treatment strategies would be required, with the criteria for minimum levels of functioning set by 'experts'. This explanation by health care providers has implications for service users on a number of levels. Firstly, the language utilised suggests a generalised approach rather than a personalised or specific one. Secondly, it looks at recovery in terms of outcomes. Thirdly, the focus is on deficits and problems as opposed to strengths and potential (Morgan, 2004). Fourthly, it suggests external treatment and monitoring have to be imposed upon service users by 'experts' in order to attain benefit. One assumes 'experts' here means health care professionals, but the term 'expert' is itself a contested concept. Barker (2003) sees health care professionals often casting themselves in the role of 'expert' by empowering themselves at the expense of the service user. Subtle phraseology can expose where the management of recovery lies. According to Altschul and Millet (2000), 'The role of psychiatry has historically been to judge the validity of patients' accounts and to correct them, via therapy' (p. xxiii).

The National Institute for Mental Health in England (NIMHE, 2004) has recommended a recovery model from the Ohio Department of Mental Health (Townsend *et al.*, 1999). The model describes how a person may be in a dependent/unaware position. At the beginning, they may have difficulty identifying needs and accepting a diagnosis, lack experience in the development of relationships, lack insight, be resistive and be totally dependent. The clinician is cast in the role of demonstrating, promoting, explaining, informing, helping, encouraging and assisting. The idioms suggest control and expertise remain with the clinician, and the service user is in a position of ignorance, lacking understanding and education and being unable to take control and to comprehend complicated aspects of medication.

Arguably, recovery should not be about meeting 'gold standards' of achievement. Neither should it be about a 'tick-box' approach in order to monitor, standardise, evaluate and organise (Blair, 2004; Kitson, 2005), which is perhaps not where policy makers and health care practitioners would wish to 'sit'. Legitimate choice may not always be afforded service users. People in receipt of services may well have different priorities from those delivering them. A top–down, one-approach-fits-all philosophy will lack flexibility and sensitivity (Mental Health Foundation, 2004). The work around recovery styles (Tait *et al.*, 2003) demonstrates the need to recognise and respect the individual response to coping and adjustment. Treatment should therefore match the recovery style. May (2001), as both a practitioner and service user, believes choice should be offered to people as to how and when they explore beliefs or whether they in fact choose to live alongside them or indeed 'seal over' (Tait *et al.*, 2003).

Perkins (2002) considers the conflict in evidence between professionals and service users, with professionals very often labelling, separating and excluding people with mental health problems and service users arguing for a right to define their own wishes and needs. Barker *et al.* (2000) state that people need fellowship as opposed to treatment and someone to join with them, as opposed to act upon them. Repper and Perkins (2003) argue that when mental difficulties are seen within the context of 'illness', they become the province of professional experts. Jacobson (2004) provides a US perspective with regard to a shift from 'power over, to power sharing' (p. 161), stating that recovery expertise occurs in the absence of professional qualifications, and is possibly only available to those with personal experience and insights. Kelly and Gamble (2005) agree that recovery can occur in the absence of professional intervention and this has the potential for creating challenging new ways of working.

Recovery does not mean that service users will cease using services or indeed become independent of services (Turner & Frak, 2001; Martyn, 2002; Perkins, 2003). What is of utmost importance is how these services are built and delivered. Repper and Perkins (2003) argue for a shift whereby recovery is not seen as a professional intervention like medication or therapy and therefore workers need to change their role from one in authority to that of coach. This is a challenge to workers who cherish the sense of power that comes with the role. Repper and Perkins (2003) furthermore refer to the need for workers to develop 'hope-inspiring relationships'. When workers struggle to work in systems that are under-resourced and when morale reaches rock-bottom, providing hope-inspiring relationships may sound a tall order. Arguably however, without this quality of relationship, it is impossible to provide the value-based care that is required to promote recovery.

Hope and optimism

The presence and need for hope is central to the recovery paradigm and there is a need for mental health workers to provide hope-inspiring relationships (Watkins, 2007; Slade, 2009). Hope is also important as it contributes to an individual's positive self-identity. Goffman (1963) proposed a theory of spoiled identities; people's identities become spoiled by society. Coping with mental health difficulties may be more manageable than the subsequent effects of stigma and discrimination. Similarly, the British Psychological Society (2000) suggests that clinical practitioners often only see those experiencing acute periods, thus getting a skewed view they describe as a 'clinician's illusion' (p. 14). This outlook can leave the clinician thinking recovery is rare and historically psychiatric provision has incorporated a fairly hopeless message. Diagnostic labels alone can have a devastating effect upon a person's sense of hope (Longden, 2001). However, the life-affirming experiences of service users do not necessarily bear out the pessimistic prognosis postulated by some stakeholders. Buckingham (2001) describes being able to relax with schizophrenia once she had overcome stigma, guilt and shame. Perkins (2001) advocates a 'normal to be different' approach.

Lester and Gask (2006) identify the enormous task of changing mental health services to become more hopeful, particularly when policies and guidance such as the NICE guidelines on schizophrenia paint a negative picture with a poor prognosis. Indeed, Barker and Buchanan-Barker (2003) question what has happened to the 'person' within the NICE guidelines on schizophrenia. They state that the guidelines are about pathology, not people, arguing that they fail to refer to peer support, the importance of recovery and the reclamation of lives or indeed the lived experience of Schizophrenia. It is therefore important not to lose the person within the milieu of guidelines.

Believing in people's potential does not require specialist professional qualification. Indeed, those general practitioners who offered encouragement and willingness to support recovery in practical ways were highly regarded in Lester *et al.*'s (2003) study. No amount of rhetoric around hope, it seems, can substitute for the reality of those actions that truly provide a catalyst for hope to flourish. These include embracing the empowerment of service users, peer support, self-help and management (Ahern & Fisher, 2001; Roberts & Wolfson, 2004; Stewart & Wheeler, 2005).

Risk and responsibility

Much of practice and policy concerns itself with risk, which is viewed differently by the stakeholder groups. The medical model offers a gloomy prognosis with emphasis on the suppression of symptoms and the safety of society (Turner & Frak, 2001). From this viewpoint, crisis should be anticipated or prevented and risk reduced (DoH, 1999). Fakhoury and Priebe (2002) argue that any government drive for safety-orientated practices will continue to alienate and stigmatise the mentally ill.

From the service-user perspective, Coleman (2011) writes of recovery requiring a degree of development, trial and error. It is also argued that recovery involves learning from experience (Turner, 2002a). If this is truly the case, practitioners who intervene to prevent difficulty may actually have a negative impact on this very process by acting as 'rescuer'. Whitehill (2003) therefore argues for a paradigm shift from that of containment to one of therapeutic experience. This involves taking risks and accepting failure (Romme & Escher, 2000; Turner, 2002a; Gould *et al.*, 2005; Coleman, 2011).

Drayton *et al.* (1998) conclude that successfully coping with psychosis is linked to a person's own subjective appraisal of it as opposed to its objective severity. Dilemmas are evident when providers attempt to 'juggle' the demands of assuming professional responsibility for risk, and the perceived protection of society with the desire to provide optimism to enable change to occur and the opportunity to nurture recovery (Stickley & Felton, 2006). Different interest groups hold different versions of any true situation. Contradictory 'truths' may lie side by side and reach consensus with differing perspectives.

There is a general consensus amongst the groups that service users ought to be central to their own recovery, that mental health services were undergoing significant changes in order to accommodate the notion of recovery and that service users must be involved in their future development and sustainability. However, tensions exist within the policy-maker and health-care practitioner groups. It also became noticeable that several factors could effectively act as 'filters' to frustrate service-user influence in their own recovery. From the intrapersonal domain, service delivery and organisation could be seen as oppositional to the personal individualistic needs; and national policy to local needs and diversity (Service Delivery and Organisation Research Development Programme, 2003). It was also noticeable that policy makers were talking in wider terms of the provision of services 'The British government's primary interest in health is with the performance, economy and acceptability of the NHS' (Baker, 2000:214), whilst service users were talking in terms of personal human experience 'I felt so miserable… not a girl anymore, just a thing' (Longden, 2001).

Service users record the experience of accepting psychosis and recovering in spite of it (Campbell, 2001). The challenge may lie in policy makers and health-care practitioners also being able to accept psychosis and to recover themselves from past patterns that may feel secure. 'Many professionals are not yet ready to think in terms of a comprehensive modern service – they are still focused on the hospital out-patient clinic-type model' (Sainsbury Centre for Mental Health, 2001:4). Again, it was not easy to know how and where these two experiences could find solidarity.

The drive for measurable and uniform services could be seen to filter out the creativity of individual expression (Turner & Frak, 2001; Blair, 2004; Kitson, 2005). The hidden influences of the pharmaceutical industry and their promotion of a biomedical model were also demonstrated by Mansfield and Jureidini (2001), and the way in which recovery is defined can act to filter and compete with the service-user experience. The service provision agenda highlighted the gulf between the biomedical perspective (defined by the elimination of symptoms) and recovery as an accepted and 'lived alongside' experience. Examples included differing messages and language concerning advice and warnings of possible long-term suffering and breakdowns and bothersome symptoms (NICE, 2002a).

Lack of hope and optimism can affect delivery of services (Longden, 2001). A pessimistic starting point is likely to frame the way in which services are provided, not only at a policy level but amongst practitioners who deliver care. Finally, issues around risk and responsibility are likely to have a direct influence on how much service users will be enabled and supported to manage and dictate the terms of their own recovery. Turner (2002a) sees this as the ability to experience one's own psychosis and develop skills in self-management.

The social construction of recovery

Social constructionists take the stance that human beings construct their world through language in different social settings. People therefore make sense of their experiences in the world through constructions of reality and meaning. Through daily interactions different frameworks of understanding and meaning are constructed from the experience. There are an unlimited number of descriptions and explanations for any form of representation, depending on the group. The construction of recovery, as already shown in this chapter, is specific and unique to the individual's experience. Each definition uses its own language and fits different disciplines, models or frameworks. It is clear that there are unlimited definitions and meanings to recovery, none of which are right or wrong, yet all unique to the individual.

However, Burr (1995) and Parker (1999) explain that the concept of social construction is not purely focused on the language used. Other important influencing factors include power and historical, cultural and social processes. Parker (1999) pulls together the issues of power and language in relation to recovery when he cites Foucault (1969) to argue:

words and phrases have meanings that are organised into systems and institutions, what Foucault (1969) called 'discursive practices' that position us in relation of power (Parker, 1999:6).

Discursive practices allow individuals to position themselves within different frameworks. The use of words such as symptoms, delusions, hallucinations and medication is essential to carry out the practice of psychiatry and similarly, for practitioners, assessments, care plans and interventions construct their reality. Without these shared words, these specific disciplines would not exist, yet these words construct our reality. As Harper (1999) explains, as soon as interventions are described as 'treatment', it 'automatically introduces a whole range of discursive positions (e.g. illness, diagnosis, recovery and cure) and a range of subject positions (e.g. of doctor and patient)' (p. 131).

The challenge for policy makers is how to avoid constructing recovery as another 'model' that practitioners work within. Whilst this may fit with the constructs and understanding of practitioners, it could destroy the essence of recovery from the service-user discourse drawn from lived experience. The challenge for the practitioner, as already discussed in this chapter, is to be able to find the meaning of recovery for the individual service user. As identified previously in this chapter, there is a risk that practitioners may 'hijack' the service-user's experience with their own discursive practices developed from day to day to clinical work and training. For example, because a person may never have heard of the concept of recovery as presented in this chapter, does not mean that he/she will not respond to a hope-inspiring relationship. In as much as the concept of recovery is understood by the worker, so the worker may construct a negotiated understanding of the concept of recovery for the person. For example, service users are all too familiar with established language within the psychiatric discourse, for example, assessment, care planning, review meetings etc. What we are suggesting therefore is that workers can (and should) contribute to a shared understanding of the concept of recovery (thus constructing meaning together), because the construct is inherently positive. Arguably far more positive than the more traditional constructs of risk assessments, care-planning compliance with medication etc. The introduction of the constructed language of recovery and a focus upon recovery concepts are intrinsically good for the client. We would also assert that this approach is intrinsically good for the worker too. For the language of recovery is inherently optimistic. So much of twenty-first century mental health care is focused upon negative constructs such as protecting the public and subsequent risk assessment. The focus of much of the Care Programme Approach is about *dis*ability, symptoms and illness. A recovery approach to care planning will focus upon wellness, the person's wishes, aspirations, hopes, plans, dreams, ideas and the resources they possess to achieve these goals.

Models for recovery

The remaining section in this chapter focuses upon specific models of mental health care that may promote recovery.

Box 3.1   Six stages to developing a wellness recovery action plan.

Section 1 – Wellness toolbox
Tools and strategies I use each day to stay well

Section 2 – Daily maintenance plan
What I do each day, when I am feeling well?

Section 3 – Dealing with triggers – External events that affect my wellness
What are my triggers and what is my response to each one/action plan.

Section 4 – Early warning signs – Internal signs/emotions that indicate changes in wellness
What are my early warning signs for me, and what is my action plan?

Section 5 – When things are breaking down – Wellness is breaking down
How do I know? Breaking down list and responses/action plan.

Section 6 – Crisis plan – To be seen by others – when I have to seek help from others
How do I know when I am well, crisis symptoms, supporters phone list, medications, treatments, treatment facilities and respite care, supporters' roles, what to do if I am in danger to myself of others, and how to know when my supports no longer need to use this plan?

(Copeland, 2001)

Wellness recovery action plan

The Wellness Recovery Action Plan (WRAP) developed by Mary-Ellen Copeland is a simple self-help tool enabling the individual to identify early warning signs, triggers and encouraging the development of coping strategies and supports. Copeland developed a WRAP from researching coping mechanisms from many of her peers. It has a resemblance to a relapse signature, which 'seeks to identify the earliest signs of impending psychotic relapse and offer timely and effective intervention' (Birchwood *et al.*, 2000:93). However, WRAP can be developed by anyone 'to relieve symptoms and/or enhance their wellness' (Copeland, 2001:127) and is completed by the individual using it and not the practitioner. The individual develops a WRAP plan, which involves working through six sections, providing guidance in developing tools, strategies and a crisis plan (see Box 3.1). The key to the plan is that the individual writes the plan entirely for him/herself, with the support of practitioners, family and friends. WRAP enables the individual to take control of their situation and have a series of plans on what to do if their wellness is not so good.

Strengths model of recovery

The Strengths Model of Recovery was developed by Charles Rapp following his frustrations regarding the culture of understanding of the human condition and how therapeutic approaches are undertaken. Perceiving an individual as 'sick' with a set of problems, abnormalities or disorders requiring professional

Box 3.2   Six principles of the strengths model.

---

1. Focus on the individual's strengths, not their weaknesses, problems or deficits;
2. The community is not an obstacle, but an oasis of resources;
3. Interventions are self-determined by the individual;
4. The Client–Practitioner relationship is the foundation of mutual collaboration;
5. Seeing the individual in their preferred environment rather than the practitioner's office;
6. Individuals with serious mental illness can continue to grow and change.

(Rapp & Goscha, 2006)

help can be disempowering and damaging. The Strengths Model takes the opposite approach to this 'Deficit Model'. It places the individual in an equal position with the professional, society and the environment, empowering them to look at their positive attributes rather than the negative.

The individual identifies their strengths, aspirations and dreams and then works towards achieving them. The aim of the practitioner is to work in collaboration with the individual to achieve the short- and long-term goals identified. Rather than using the professional discourse as a basis for the relationship; the service users own language is used to gather information, to undertake a strengths assessment and to identify useful and supportive resources within the wider community (Rapp & Goscha, 2006). Box 3.2 illustrates the six principles of the Strengths Model.

Tidal model

The Tidal Model, developed by Phil Barker in the UK, drew on the theoretical work of Peplau (1952) and also from research (by Chris Stevenson and Sue Jackson) which explored what people need mental health nurses for. The philosophy of the model is based on six principles (Box 3.3). It focuses on how personal experience and human needs form and create new narratives which

Box 3.3   Six principles of the Tidal Model.

---

1. Curiosity – The professional knows nothing about the person and his/her experience. The individual is the expert of their experience and the role of the practitioner is to explore the individual's experience with curiosity;
2. Resourcefulness – Instead of focusing on diagnosis, symptoms or illness, the individual is encouraged to focus on their resources, using a solutions-focused approach;
3. Respect for the person's wishes – The role of the practitioner is to take the individual's wishes seriously;
4. Crisis as an opportunity – A crisis is seen as an opportunity for change, rethink life path and do something differently, rather than seeing a crisis as something to cope with or control;
5. Think small – Following the solution-focused approach, individuals are encouraged to take small steps forward and not set big, less-achievable goals;
6. Elegance – Care plans are simple, with simple interventions.

(Barker, 2000)

allow the sense of self that has been lost through trauma and everyday distress to be restored. The model acknowledges the fluid nature of human experience:

Life is a journey undertaken on an ocean of experience. All human developments, including the experience of illness and health, involve discoveries made on the journey across that ocean of experience (Barker, 2001:235).

Recovery values and implementation

The models, philosophies and approaches to recovery presented here all have similar themes running through them. This emphasises that recovery is a set of values or attitude that practitioners need to adopt rather than a prescriptive model. By placing the concept of recovery within a box, as illustrated in Box 3.1, Box 3.2 and Box 3.3, it may make the practitioners work easier but could destroy the essence of recovery. Simply implementing any of these models would not achieve 'recovery' as the human experience is so fluid and complex; instead, practitioners need to have a number of tools and values which are adaptable to the individual's needs and beliefs. This leads to the question of whether an effective recovery-orientated service can be integrated within the current mental health system. As previously mentioned within this chapter, recovery cannot stand alone within mental health services and there still needs to be large changes in organisational culture for recovery values and principles to be fully embedded. We have already highlighted that the ImRoC project (Boardman & Shepherd, 2012) is evaluating the use of a framework to implement recovery within six demonstration sites in the UK. This framework presents ten key challenges that need to be addressed by mental health services if they are to move towards becoming recovery orientated. These are listed in the following:

- Changing the nature of day-to-day interactions and the quality of experience;
- Delivering comprehensive, user-led education and training programmes;
- Establishing a 'recovery education unit' to drive the programmes forward;
- Ensuring organisational commitment, creating the culture. The importance of leadership;
- Increasing personalisation and choice;
- Changing the way we approach risk assessment and management;
- Redefining user involvement;
- Transforming the workforce;
- Supporting staff in their recovery journey;
- Increasing opportunities for building a life 'beyond illness'.

The ImRoC project presents an exciting opportunity within the UK for developing a whole systems approach to the delivery of recovery-orientated mental health services. However, the project is on-going and the findings have not yet been reported. Elsewhere in the world, there are existing recovery-orientated services which can be learnt from. As well as the organisational approach taken by ImRoC, there are examples of good practice of individual service areas within organisations which work to promote recovery. One such example is a recovery-orientated acute mental health service in New Zealand.

A similar organisation is ICRA-WholeLife (see www.icra-wholelife.org), which has been introduced earlier in this chapter. Drawing on education, research and practice ICRA aims to provide a platform for anyone to embed recovery into practice. Recovery is not just for mental health services, but for all aspects of life.

Recovery-orientated acute mental health service

The Capital and Coast Home Based Treatment service within New Zealand has adopted a philosophy that although people experiencing a crisis are in danger, they are also presented with an opportunity. By working in partnership as a collaborative approach with the service user, clinician and family, the crisis can be turned to an opportunity for self-determination, self-efficiency and an opportunity for personal growth, whilst still minimising risks (Goldsack *et al.*, 2005). The service does not act as a replacement to hospital treatment, rather an alternative, providing the individual with a choice of support. The team encourages an open and transparent communication policy involving the family and partners. By taking this stance, privacy issues are avoided and the risk of power imbalances reduced. Once open communication is formed, families and individuals can develop trust in the team and levels of distress decrease. The team works to encourage the individual in crisis to identify how they can be helped. This enables the practitioner to give simple levels of caring and facilitates a connection with the individual and their family/partner.

The New Zealand Mental Health Commission published a report evaluating this service to see if what it offered was recovery orientated. Using a narrative approach, Goldsack *et al.* (2005) found that service users and families were very positive in the way they were offered practical help, advice and information. Visits, often several times a day, provided reassurance and support, as the team formed strong supportive relationships to both service user and their family. People felt they were treated as individuals, and included in decisions with hope and encouragement of recovery. Team members were also very positive about their work, with their nursing skills being drawn upon, clearly being able to articulate a recovery philosophy (Goldsack *et al.*, 2005).

Recovery outcome measurement tools

In recent years, there has been a growth of outcome measurement tools. Two more well-used tools in the UK are the Scottish Recovery Indicator and the Recovery Star. In other countries, tools include Developing Recovery Enhancing Environments Measure (DREEM) and Ohio Consumer

Assessment. For many, the idea of measuring recovery could lead to it becoming institutionalised within services, and recovery becoming defined by services and not the individual. However, in a culture of outcomes- and evidence-based practice, recovery needs to be measured to satisfy the needs of service providers. Tools are in their infancy, yet perhaps a way forward would be in developing one which also acts to aid people's recovery.

Conclusion

In this chapter, we have explored the complex world of recovery by considering the social construction of recovery and its historical developments. By analysing recent literature, we have identified key themes relating to the subject. We have looked at models of recovery and considered how the mental health worker might authentically work within such models whilst retaining their integrity. For some people who have used mental health services over a period of years, the language of service providers has affected them. They may see themselves as 'hopeless'. Working in a recovery-promoting way may be hard for the person to accept. There are those that may no longer be confined within the brick walls of the asylums, but psychologically have become institutionalised to the psychiatric discourse. For they may see little hope for themselves beyond reduction of symptoms by changing medication. A challenge to mental health workers who wish to work within a recovery paradigm is to let the client define what recovery means to them, and to use their language. It is all too easy to restrict people by our own language and approach.

The individual worker will need to decide for oneself if it is possible to work with individuals towards recovery without destroying the concept. We argue that it is possible, but this largely depends upon the worker's willingness to listen to the person's hopes, dreams and aspirations and genuinely work with the person to achieve these. Understanding of mental health problems needs to go way beyond the biomedical definitions and approaches. For much of what we refer to today as 'mental illness' is more to do with the pathology of society than the pathology of the person.

It can be argued that services require a degree of structure and organisation in order to deliver quality care and retain accountability to public funds. Despite this, it will be important for those who provide these services to be able to demonstrate flexibility, which includes being able to effect any necessary paradigm shift (Sainsbury Centre for Mental Health, 2001). Workers will need to believe that recovery is possible (Kelly & Gamble, 2005) and accept a shift in authority to that of working 'alongside' (Repper & Perkins, 2003). To work with a recovery philosophy in mind will require workers to allow service users to define recovery for themselves and to work collaboratively with the service-users' own style. This is likely to throw up dilemmas for workers with implications at policy level, not least in the domain of risk taking.

We acknowledge that there is currently a fear amongst many people that recovery will be destroyed and 'colonised' by professionals, becoming another thing done to them. It is our hope that this chapter has not contributed to that problem. What we have endeavoured to demonstrate is that the positive construction of recovery can be used as a vehicle for good practice. Arguably, unless the workers have experienced mental health problems themselves, the true essence of recovery cannot be captured. However, with a change in attitude and approach to a belief that there is hope for the seemingly hopeless, that there are endless opportunities for change and growth, the careful art of care planning can be part of a person's journey to recovery.

I cannot think of anything more destructive to one's sense of worth as a human being than to believe that the inner core of one's being is sick – that one's thoughts, values, feelings and beliefs are merely the meaningless thoughts, values, feelings, and beliefs are merely the meaningless symptoms of a sick mind (Modrow, 1996:147).

References

Ahern, L. & Fisher, D. (2001) Recovery at your own pace. *Journal of Psychosocial Nursing and Mental Health Services*, **39** (4), 22–32.

Altschul, A. & Millet, K. (2000) Forward. In: *From the Ashes of Experience: Reflections on Madness, Survival and Growth* (eds P. Barker, P. Campbell & B. Davidson). pp. xi–xv. Whurr Publishers, London.

Baker, M. (2000) *Making Sense of the NHS White Papers*, 2nd edn. Radcliffe Medical Press, Oxon.

Barchard, C. (2005) *Voices Forum* [online]. Available at http://www.voicesforum.org.uk/ideasma.htm. Accessed on November 22, 2005.

Barker, P. (2000) Turning the tide. *Open Mind*, **106**, 10–11.

Barker, P. (2001) The tidal model: developing an empowering, person centred approach to recovery within psychiatric and mental health nursing. *Journal of Psychiatric and Mental Health Nursing*, **8** (3), 233–240.

Barker, P. (2003) The primacy of caring. Cited In: *Psychiatric and Mental Health Nursing: The Craft of Caring* (ed P. Barker). pp. 607–618. Arnold, London.

Barker, P. & Buchanan-Barker, P. (2003) Not so NICE guidelines. *Open Mind*, **121**, 14.

Barker, P. Campbell, P. & Davidson, B. (2000) *From the Ashes of Experience: Reflections on Madness, Survival and Growth*. Whurr Publishers, London.

Birchwood, M. Spencer, E. & McGovern, D. (2000) Schizophrenia: early warning signs. *Advance in Psychiatric Treatment*, **6**, 93–101.

Blair, G. (2004) The new GMS contract and its implications for mental health. *Community Mental Health*, **3** (2), 12–14.

Boardman, J. & Shepherd, G. (2012) *Implementing Recovery Through Organisational Change (ImROC)* [Online]. Available at http://www.centreformentalhealth.org.uk/recovery/supporting_recovery.aspx. Accessed on May 27, 2013.

Bonney, S. & Stickley, T. (2008) Recovery and mental health: a review of the British literature. *Journal of Psychiatric and Mental Health Nursing*, **15** (2), 140–153.

British Psychological Society (2000) *Recent Advances in Understanding Mental Illness and Psychotic Experiences*. Division of Clinical Psychologists, Leicester.

Buckingham, C. (2001) Schizophrenia – the biological and social. *Open Mind*, **111**, 11.

Burr, V. (1995) *An Introduction to Social Constructionism*. Routledge, London.

Campbell, P. (2001) It's not the real you. *Open Mind*, **111**, 16–17.

Campbell, J. & Gallagher, R. (2007) *A Literature Review and Documentary Analysis on Recovery Training in Mental Health Practice* [Online]. Available from AskClyde at www.scottishrecovery.net/…/94-Recovery-Training-Review.html. Accessed on May 6, 2013.

Carless, D. & Douglas, K. (2008) Narrative, identity and mental health: how men with serious mental illness re-story their lives through sport and exercise. *Psychology of Sport and Exercise*, **9** (5), 576–594.

Chalmers, F. (2001) *Psychiatry 'Hijacked' by Big Pharma* [Online]. Available at http://healthmatters.org.uk/issue45/bigpharma. Accessed on July 7, 2006.

Coleman, R. (2011) *Recovery: An Alien Concept*. P&P Press, Isle of Lewis.

Coleman, R., Baker, P. & Taylor, K. (2001) *Working to Recovery, Victim to Victor: A Guide to Mental Wellbeing, a Personal Planning Tool*. Handsell Publishing, Gloucester.

Copeland, M. E. (2001) Wellness recovery action plan: a system for monitoring, reducing and eliminating uncomfortable or dangerous psychical symptoms and emotional feelings. *Occupational Therapy in Mental Health*, **17** (3/4), 5–21.

Copeland, M. E. (2006) *Mental Health Recovery and Wellness Recovery Action Plan (WRAP)* [Online]. Available at http://www.mentalhealthrecovery.com/about/overview.php. Accessed on May 27, 2013.

Deegan, P. (1993) Recovering our sense of value after being labelled mentally ill. *Journal of Psychosocial Nursing*, **31** (4), 7–11.

Deegan, P. (2001) Recovery as a self-directed process of healing and transformation. *Occupational Therapy Mental Health*, **17** (3–4), 5–21.

Department of Health (DoH) (1983) *The Mental Health Act 1983*. Stationery Office, London.

Department of Health (1999) *A National Service Framework for Mental Health. Modern Standards and Service Models*. Stationery Office, London.

Department of Health (2001) *The Journey to Recovery – the Government's Vision for Mental Health Care*. Stationery Office, London.

Department of Health (2002) *Developing Services for Carers and Families of People with Mental Illness*. Stationery Office, London.

Department of Health (2003) *Continuity of Care for People with Severe Mental Illness* [Online]. Service Delivery and Organisation Research Development Programme. Briefing Paper. Available at http://www.netscc.ac.uk/hsdr/files/project/SDO_BP_08-1109-009_V01.pdf. Accessed on May 27, 2013.

Department of Health (2005) *New Ways of Working for Psychiatrists: Enhancing Effective, Person-Centred Services Through New Ways of Working in Multidisciplinary and Multi-agency Contexts*. Royal College of Psychiatrists, National Institute for Mental Health in England and Changing Workforce Programme, London.

Department of Health (2009) *NICE Guidelines: Schizophrenia: Core Interventions in the Treatment and Management of Schizophrenia in Adults in Primary and Secondary Care*. The Stationery Office, London.

Department of Health & Hope, R. (2004) *The Ten Essential Shared Capabilities – a Framework for the Whole of the Mental Health Workforce.* Stationery Office, London.

Drayton, M., Birchwood, M. & Trower, P. (1998) Early attachment experiences and recovery from psychosis. *British Journal of Clinical Psychology,* **37,** 269–284.

Fakhoury, W. & Priebe, S. (2002) The process of deinstitutionalisation: an international overview. *Current Opinion in Psychiatry,* **15** (2) 187–192.

Fisher, D. (2000) Hope, humanity and voice in recovery from mental illness. Cited in: *From the Ashes of Experience. Reflections on Madness, Survival and Growth* (eds P. Barker, P. Campbell & B. Davidson). Whurr Publishers, London.

Fisher, D. (2005) *A New Vision of Recovery: People can fully Recover from Mental Illness; It is not a Life-long Process* [Online]. Available at http://www.power2u.org/who.html. Accessed on April 29, 2013.

Foucault, M. (1969) *The Archaeology of Knowledge.* Tavistock, London.

Goffman, E. (1963) *Stigm a: Notes on the Management of Spoiled Identity.* Pelican Books, London.

Goldsack, S., Reet, M., Lapsley, H. & Gingell, M. (2005) *Experiencing a Recovery-Orientated Acute Mental Health Service: Home Based Treatment from the Perspectives of Service Users, their Families and Mental Health Professionals.* Mental Health Commission, Wellington, New Zealand.

Gould, A., DeSouza, S. & Rebeiro-Gruhl, K. (2005) And then I lost that life: a shared narrative of four young men with schizophrenia. *British Journal of Occupational Therapy,* **68** (10), 467–473.

Grierson, M. (2001) *Emerging Best Practice in Mental Health: User-based Outcomes and Recovery* [Online]. Available at http://www.mhrecovery.com/components.htm. Accessed on May 27, 2013.

Harper, D. (1999) Tablet talk and deport discourse: discourse analysis and psychiatric medication. In: *Applied Discourse Analysis: Social and Psychological Interventions* (ed Willig, C.). pp. 124–144. Open University Press, Buckingham.

Harrison, G., Hopper, K., Craig, T., *et al.* (2001) Recovery from psychotic illness: a 15 and 25 year international follow up study. *The British Journal of Psychiatry,* **178,** 506–517.

Heather, F. (2002) Pro-motion: a positive way forward for clients with severe and enduring mental health problems living in the community, Part 1. *British Journal of Occupational Therapy,* **65** (12), 551–558.

Holloway, F. (2002) Outcome measurement in mental health. Welcome to the revolution. *The British Journal of Psychiatry,* **181,** 1–2.

Jacobson, N. (2004) *In Recovery: The Making of Mental Health Policy.* Vanderbilt University Press, Nashville.

Kelly, M. & Gamble, C. (2005) Exploring the concept of recovery in schizophrenia. *Journal of Psychiatric and Mental Health Nursing,* **12** (2), 245–251.

Kendell, R.E. (2000) The next 25 years. *The British Journal of Psychiatry,* **176,** 6–9.

Kitson, C. (2005) Roads to recovery. *Mental Health Today,* **May,** 16.

Leamy, M., Bird, V., Le Boutillier, C., Williams, J. & Slade, M. (2011) Conceptual framework for personal recovery in mental health: systematic review and narrative synthesis. *The British Journal of Psychiatry,* **199,** 445–452.

Lester, H. & Gask, L. (2006) Delivering medical care for patients with serious mental illness or promoting a collaborative model of recovery. *British Journal of Psychiatry,* **188,** 401–402.

Lester, H., Tritter, J. & England, E. (2003) Satisfaction with primary care: the perspectives of people with schizophrenia. *Family Practice* **20** (5), 508–513.

Lester, H., Tritter, J, & Sorohan, H. (2005) Patients' and health professionals' views on primary care for people with serious mental illness: focus group study. *British Medical Journal*, **330**, 1122.

Longden, E. (2001) Suspended animation. *Open Mind*, **111**, 12–13.

MacDonald, A. (2005) *Milestones on My Recovery Road* [Online]. Available from Scottish Recovery Network at http://www.scottishrecovery.net. Accessed on May 6, 2013.

Mansfield, P. & Jureidini, J. (2001) *Giving Doctors the Treatment* [Online]. Available at http://healthmatters.org.uk/issue43/givingdoctors. Accessed on May 6, 2013.

Martyn, D. (2002) *The Experiences and Views of Self Management of People with a Schizophrenia Diagnosis*. Rethink, London.

May, R. (2000a) Psychosis & Recovery. *Open Mind*, **106**, 24–25.

May, R. (2000b) Routes to recovery from psychosis: the roots of a clinical psychologist. *Clinical Psychology Forum*, **146**, 6–10.

May, R. (2001) *Understanding Psychotic Experience and Working Towards Recovery*. Bradford District Community Trust, Bradford.

May, R., Risman, J., Kidder, K., *et al.* (1999) *Recovery Advisory Group Recovery Model. A Work in Process* [Online]. Available from Recovery Advisory Group at www.mhsip.org/recovery/index.html. Accessed on May 27, 2013].

Mead S. & Copeland M.E. (2000) What recovery means to us: consumers' perspective. *Community Mental Health Journal*, **36** (3), 315–328.

Mental Health Foundation (2004) *Response to Consultation Document – New Vision for Adult Social Care (SCIE 2004)* [Online]. Available at www.mentalhealth.org.uk. Accessed on November 21, 2005.

Modrow, J. (1996) *How to Become a Schizophrenic*, Apollyon Press, Washington.

Morgan, S. (2004) Strengths based practice. *Open Mind*, **126**, 16–17.

National Institute for Clinical Excellence (NICE) (2002a) *Treating and Managing Schizophrenia (Core Interventions) Understanding NICE Guidance Information for People with Schizophrenia, their Advocates and Carers and the Public*. NICE, London.

National Institute for Clinical Excellence (2002b) *Core Interventions in the Treatment and Management of Schizophrenia in Primary and Secondary Care. Clinical Practice Algorithms and Pathways to Care*. NICE, London.

National Institute for Clinical Excellence & National Collaborating Centre for Mental Health (2003) *Full National Clinical Guideline on Core Interventions in Primary and Secondary Care*. Gaskell and British Psychological Society, London.

National Institute for Mental Health in England (NIMHE) (2003) *Recovery and Change – Mental Health into the Mainstream*. NIMHE/DoH, Leeds.

National Institute for Mental Health in England (2004) *Emerging Best Practice in Mental Health Recovery*. NIMHE/DoH, Leeds.

National Institute for Mental Health in England (2005) *Making it Possible: Improving Mental Health and Well-being in England*. NIMHE/DoH, Leeds.

Nolan, P. (2000) History of psychiatry, patients and hospitals. *Current opinion in psychiatry*, **13** (6), 717–720.

Parker, I (1999) *Critical Textwork: An Introduction to Varieties of Discourse and Analysis*. Open University Press, Buckingham.

Peplau, H. E. (1952) *Interpersonal Relations in Nursing*. Putman, New York.

Perkins, R. (2001) Stigma or discrimination. *Open Mind*, **112**, 6.

Perkins, R. (2002) The right to define reality. *Open Mind*, **116**, 14.

Perkins, R. (2003) The altar of independence. *Open Mind*, **119**, 6.

Rapp, C. A. & Goscha R. J. (2006) *The Strengths Model: Case Management with People with Psychiatric Disabilities*. Oxford University Press, Oxford.

Reid, Y., Johnson, S., Bebbington, P., Kuipers, E., Scott, H. & Thornicroft, G. (2001) The longer term outcomes of community care: a 12 year follow-up of the Camberwell high contact survey. *Psychological Medicine*, **31** (2), 351–359.

Repper, J. & Ford, R. (2006) How can nurses build trusting relationships with people who have severe and long term mental health problems? Experiences of case managers and their clients. *Journal of Advanced Nursing*, **19** (6), 1096–1104.

Repper, J. & Perkins, R. (2003) *Social Inclusion and Recovery: A Model for Mental Health Practice*. Bailliere Tindall, London.

Repper, J. & Perkins, R. (2009) Recovery and social inclusion. In: *Mental Health Nursing Skills* (eds P. Callaghan, J. Playle & L. Cooper). pp. 85–95. Oxford University Press, Oxford.

Rethink (2005) *Recovery – A Brief Introduction to the Recovery Approach* [Online]. Available at http://www.rethink.org/recovery. Accessed on April 29, 2013].

Roberts, G. & Wolfson, P. (2004) The rediscovery of recovery: open to all. *Advances in Psychiatric Treatment*, **10** (1), 37–48.

Roberts, G., Dorkins, E., Wooldridge, J. & Hewis, E. (2008) Detained – What's my choice? A discussion paper. *Advances in Psychiatric Treatment*, **14**, 183–184.

Romme, M. & Escher, S. (2000) *Making Sense of Voices*. Mind Publications, London.

Sainsbury Centre for Mental Health (2001) *Mental Health Policy: The Challenges Facing the Government*. SCMH, London.

Sayce, L. (2000) *From Psychiatric Patient to Citizen*. Macmillan Press, Basingstoke.

Service Delivery and Organisation Research Development Programme & National Health Service (2003) *Continuity of Care for People with Severe Mental Illness?* SDORD, London.

Slade, M. (2009) *Personal Recovery and Mental Illness: A Guide for Mental Health Professionals*. Cambridge University Press, Cambridge.

Spandler, H., Secker, J., Kent, L., Hacking, S. & Shenton, J. (2007) Catching life: the contribution of arts initiatives to recovery approaches in mental health. *Journal of Psychiatric and Mental Health Nursing*, **14** (8), 791–799.

Stanton, S. (2001) Inescapable past? *Open Mind*, **111**, 15.

Stewart, L. & Wheeler, K. (2005) Occupation for recovery. *Occupational Therapy News*, **13** (11), 20.

Stickley, T. & Felton, A. (2006) Promoting recovery through therapeutic risk taking. *Mental Health Practice*, **9** (8), 26–30.

Stickley, T. & Wright, N. (2011a) The British research evidence for recovery, papers published between 2006–2009 (inclusive). Part One: A review of the peer-reviewed literature using a systematic approach. *Journal of Psychiatric and Mental Health Nursing*, **18** (3), 247–256.

Stickley, T. & Wright, N. (2011b) The British research evidence for recovery, papers published between 2006–2009 (inclusive). Part Two: A review of the grey literature including book chapters and policy documents. *Journal of Psychiatric and Mental Health Nursing*, **8** (4), 297–307.

Tait, L., Birchwood, M. & Trower, P. (2003) Predicting engagement with services for psychosis: insight, symptoms and recovery style. *The British Journal of Psychiatry*, **182**, 123–128.

Townsend, W., Boyd, S., Griffin, G. & Hicks, P. (1999) *Emerging Best Practices in Mental Health Recovery*. Ohio Department of Mental Health, Columbus.

Travis, M., Peters, E. & Kerwin, R. (2001) *Managing Relapse in Schizophrenia*. Science Press Ltd, London.

Turner, D. (2002a) Mapping the routes to recovery. *Mental Health Today*, **July**, 29–30.

Turner, D. (2002b) The national voices forum. Cited in: *The Regaining Control Conference*. National Voices Forum and UK Advocacy Network, Oxford.

Turner, D. & Frak, D. (2001) *Wild Geese: Recovery in National Schizophrenia Fellowship*. Green Gauge Consultancy and NSF Wales, Powys.

Warner, R. (2004) *Recovery from Schizophrenia*, 3rd edn. Brunner-Routledge, Hove.

Watkins, P.N. (2007) *Recovery: A Guide for Mental Health Practitioners*. Churchill Livingstone, London.

Whitehill, I. (2003) The concept of recovery. Cited in: *Psychiatric and Mental Health Nursing: The Craft of Caring* (ed P. Barker) pp. 43–49. Arnold, London.

Wimberley, L. & Peters, A. (2003) Recovery in acute mental health. *Occupational Therapy News*, **July**, 25.

World Health Organization (WHO) (2005) *Mental Health Declaration for Europe. Facing the Challenges, Building Solutions* [Online]. Available at http://www.euro.who.int/__data/assets/pdf_file/0008/88595/E85445.pdf. Accessed on May 27, 2013.

Section 1

Surviving

Chapter 4

Discovering the Person

Angela Hall and Donna Piper

Teesside University, UK

Understanding the perspective of another person is essential if we are to be able to put our expertise at the disposal of that individual in a constructive way (Repper & Perkins, 2003:21)

Introduction

How can we ever come to know someone? Pondering on who could ever claim to know me, the full me, then the answer would be no-one, as I allow only some pieces of myself be known to certain people. Some people may claim to know me or judge me but they do so without all of the necessary information or insight into my life and my world. What would it take for me to allow someone, not just anyone to fully know me and my lived experiences? This is perhaps the question we need to ask ourselves as we set out to enter someone else's world, often someone who is experiencing some level of psychological distress. So it is perhaps naive and disrespectful to think that we can in any encounters come to 'know' the complexity and dynamism of that person. Probably, the best we can ever hope to achieve is a shared view of the person's distress, and how they would like to be helped or supported. It is acknowledged that when working towards recovery and prior to planning care for people experiencing any form of mental illness, it is essential to have an understanding of the person's experiences/situation. It is also the starting point of any therapeutic involvement and sets the foundation for the future development of the person's interaction with professional services.

This chapter aims to explore the process of assessment within the care planning process but hopefully within the context of a person's recovery and examine some of the implications for the mental health practitioner (MHP) and their practice. The term assessment raises issues for those attempting to

Care Planning in Mental Health: Promoting Recovery, Second Edition.
Edited by Angela Hall, Michael Wren and Stephan D. Kirby.
© 2013 John Wiley & Sons, Ltd. Published 2013 by John Wiley & Sons, Ltd.

adopt a more recovery-focused approach as historically and organisationally, and assessment is done by the 'experts' to others. However, this chapter will identify how by a change in approach the assessment process can be humanised by practitioners to shape and improve the experience for people and how despite the medicalisation and bureaucracy within mental health care, they can come to know people in a more meaningful, person-focused way.

When we attempt to make sense of and understand a person's experience of mental distress, we begin on a journey of discovery. Whether assessment is the right term for this journey, in which one person learns about another, how they have experienced life, what their dreams and desires are as well as their ghosts and demons, is debatable. According to the American Psychological Association, the term assessment is defined as 'assess. (nd): to judge or estimate the value, character, etc of...' (APA, 2007).

It is something that everyone is familiar with, we assess everything constantly – what brand of baked beans to buy; which car will be the best; when is it safe to cross the road? However, when we use the word assess in relation to mental distress, it can be perceived as very clinical and professional where one person judges the worth of another or makes judgements regarding that person's ability. This approach reinforces a medical model and is based on professional power/expertise, the expert from the assessment decides what is wrong with the person and decides how this can be put right. The use of a structured framework and/or an outcome-focused assessment tool can reinforce this position of the professional having the expertise and the right questions to ask and setting the agenda for the interaction. Using this approach, it can become ritualistic as the professional becomes more familiar and more staid with the process and questions, which limits the opportunity for a more collaborative, person-centred exploration of the person's distress.

The common practice of MHPs to also focus on a person's symptoms or problems can often leave the person feeling negative and hopeless about themselves and their lives. Repper and Perkins (2003) warn MHPs of the 'limits of our expertise' (p. 13) and encourage us to 'listen to people with mental health problems' (p. 14). It sounds simple, and most professionals would argue that they do listen, so why then do service users and carers continue to report that 'they never listen'? (Lindow, 1996:14).

Watkins (2001) emphasises the need for practitioners to gain a more balanced view of the person by also valuing the richer narratives that they can offer including their qualities, strengths and achievements. This in turn can lead to a more hope inspiring perspective. 'This is where assessment and recovery become interwoven in the helping process' (Watkins, 2001:59). It is important that MHPs are not entrenched in the historically pessimistic view of mental illness as a lifelong illness in which there will be many relapses and resulting disabilities, as this view will stifle any belief in recovery or the hope that people can adapt, change or improve their lives. People in recovery can generally identify the incident that turned around their lives, and it is often linked to someone who treats them 'differently', enabling them to see other possibilities. Deegan (1988) describes this as 'the loving invitation to be something more' (p. 14).

This discourse is compatible with the concept of recovery and the promotion of collaborative working. If we deconstruct the word assessment, in terms of human interaction, it is a relationship in which one person facilitates the other to tell their story. It is how we come to 'see' the person as they present to us, what they choose or sometimes do not choose to tell us. But to 'see' we need to 'look', but it is how we do this that can influence what we 'see'. If we are looking for problems and difficulties, we will find them; if we look for risk factors, we will find them; if we look for symptoms or a diagnosis, we will find them.

So, our point is that much of what we look for as MHPs is constrained by a system with a dominant medical/social control discourse. This has been further compounded, as much of today's evidence-based practice (i.e., via NICE) is constructed to guide MHP in relation to best practice for people with depression, anxiety and schizophrenia, to name but a few. It has become so internalised that often we are unaware of how omnipotent it is when we meet people and how this can create an environment of destructive, dehumanising and stigmatising encounters.

How then do we unburden ourselves from the organisational, professional and theoretical shackles? The answer is honestly, we cannot as it is currently, the world in which we live and to do so could lead to chaos and destruction; however, as MHPs, we can shield people from the disabling effects of the system by relating to them differently, by seeing them as unique individuals with similar needs and desires common to all. The underpinning values needed to enable a person's recovery are essentially humanistic, with its roots in phenomenology, it does not seek to theorise or label a person's experience; rather, it serves to make sense or understand the person's behaviour in relation to their lived experiences, their subjective world. Hence we begin to understand the person and not the 'label', and this involves MHP seeing the person first and not being influenced by any label, seeing the person with very individual needs, strengths and aspirations.

Any information gathered is collaborative and forms the basis of a shared understanding and explanation of the person's world. In mental health, it is mainly subjective and relies on the person being able to disclose the information. To assess means to make a judgement about, but what judgements are we trying to make, is it in relation to their illness, their ability or inability, problems, strengths or weaknesses? It is all of these and more as we are trying to put together a jigsaw that represents the whole person, but often without all of the pieces.

Box 4.1   Areas for consideration during an assessment.

- Previous history/life map;
- Previous family relationships;
- Previous illness – physical/mental;
- Education and work history/aspirations;
- Current relationship, family and support networks;
- Child care/child protection issues;
- Housing/finance and benefits;
- Neighbourhood and community networks – if any;
- Religion/spiritual/cultural issues of importance;
- Physical health needs;
- Hygiene, diet and lifestyle;
- Services used currently or in the past as well as the service;
- User's and carer's views about these services;
- Any experiences that may be considered risky;
- Psychological experiences/presenting issues;
- What are their personal goals and aspirations;
- What ways of coping are being used already;
- Disengaging/terminating the interview.

Gathering the information is not a one-off process although at times it can be presented as such, often referred to in practice as *the* assessment (Box 4.1), this is often reinforced by the subsequent documentation involved. The initial contact with a person is often the beginning of this ongoing process, which leads to the discovery of various pieces of information, which help build up a detailed picture of the person. As each new piece of information is received (added), then this contributes to the 'decision making process' (Barker, 1997:6).

The aim of assessing someone's mental health is to enable the person, and the people involved in their care gain insight and understanding of the person's lived experience. This enables the person to be involved and be an active partner in the care planning process. So assessment should not be done to people; rather, it should be done with people in a collaborative way.

The process of finding out about another person is generally on-going in that the MHP is continuously observing for any changes or additional information to help in the understanding of a person's distress. This is vital as even the smallest of detail can indicate a change in the person's mood or thinking having potential impact on their behaviour. Each time the MHP engages with the person, on each contact or at each visit, they are alert to that interaction and the meaning and value of it. Initially, the MHP will be aiming to gather a broad overview of the person's situation and issues; it is about assessing the whole person or whole phenomenon. This can be achieved by engaging in a collaborative dialogue in which the person is encouraged to explore and reflect on different aspects of their lives, by encouraging the person to lead this; it ensures that issues important to them are identified, rather than the MHP setting the areas for discussion; however, it may be that the person feels lost and unable to converse in which case the MHP may need to facilitate and prompt the discussion. This type of information is often termed as subjective in that it is the person's perspective of their lives, their story and thus has meaning to them. The word subjective in scientific and evidence-based approaches often has negative connotations as it is not considered as 'accurate' or 'reliable' as objective information. So, again, the MHPs need to challenge this notion and recognise the strength of a person's narrative. It is as Barker (2000) acknowledges, 'their words, their story'. It would be this rich and meaningful information that would be valued with a recovery-orientated approach as in Barker's Tidal Model.

The information needed to gain a real understanding of the person's situation can be gained from a variety of methods as identified by Barker (1997):

- Questionnaires and rating scales;
- Direct observation;
- Logs, diaries and records;
- Interviewing.

Questionnaires and rating scales

There are many standardised tools that aim to quantify a persons' overall, symptomatology such as the Krawiecka, Goldberg and Vaughn (KGV) assessment scale (Krawiecka *et al.*, 1977) or overall Quality of Life (Priebe *et al.*, 1999). Clarifying or more specific assessments can focus on particular aspects of the person's life or experience that has been identified during the global (overall) assessment. These assessments allow a deeper exploration of a single issue. For example, measuring distress relating to delusional ideas or investigating the consistency of family relationships and support. The majority of standardised assessment tools have been developed from research. Therefore, they are tried and tested to ensure that they are valid and reliable tools. Tools have been developed to measure both global and specific aspects of mental health, and Gamble and Brennan (2000) have developed a useful glossary of some of the key assessment tools for people with serious mental illness. Choosing and using the most appropriate assessments can lead to an enhancement of the collaborative process as both the person and the MHP search for meaning. 'Using and choosing appropriate assessments is the foundation on which successful, collaborative intervention is built' (p. 3).

They attempt to provide a quantifiable measure of a particular area such as anxiety or depression levels as well as measuring overall functioning or symptomatology. The use of such tools has inherent difficulties, as they tend to compartmentalise aspects of complex human behaviour that is then quantified leaving the assessor to tick the correct box. The approach by the MHP when utilising such tools is paramount, in ensuring that it is introduced as a useful and relevant tool for the person and the benefits it can offer in relation to understanding the person's experience and is done in a collaborative way rather than as the expert doing to the person.

In social work, there is a wealth of tools supporting assessment – the Framework for the Assessment of Children in **Need and their Families**, which was first published by DoH (2000), is the document followed when assessing children and their families. Adult social care utilise the single assessment tool; however, it is vital that the assessment process in either needs to be person-led and undertaken in collaboration with the individual and to focus on the individual strengths and resilience. In essence, focusing on what a person can do and work with the skill base that is already in place. It is essential that the assessment process incorporates the individual's social, community and family support networks.

In some cases, the actual method of assessment that is used is determined by the person; for instance, it may be that some people could become anxious and agitated with any of the earlier methods or tools. In our experience, however, it is often with the more complex and comprehensive assessment tools like KGV (Krawiecka *et al.*, 1977) that it is more likely to happen. Therefore, it is important to begin with an approach that will encourage the engagement process and encourage the person to express their perspective. The assessment method must be relevant to the person being assessed, and it is also important that they understand the rationale and purpose of the method being used (Barker, 1997).

Direct observation

By observing a person, the MHP can gain valuable information about the person sometimes it may be information that the person is not consciously aware of but is being demonstrated in their nonverbal communication. Observation skills can be used generally or more specifically (Trevithick, 2005). However, it is often a neglected method, and the relevance of observations is often ignored. By rigorous observations of the person, a pattern of behaviour can be identified and shared with the person to enhance understanding of their experiences.

Observations can be made by:

- Any involved practitioner;
- Relevant others, family, friends and carers;
- The person themselves.

(Barker, 1997)

The frequency and duration of certain behaviours can be measured and noted, that is, how often and for how long a person spends talking to nonexistent voices. Self-monitoring is a useful way of involving the person more actively in the assessment process and helping them to understand the connections between thoughts, feelings and behaviours. Following on from the initial assessment, together with the MHP, they can agree what behaviours, thoughts or feelings are to be recorded. The person may agree to count the number of times they experience a specific thought, feeling or behaviour (frequency). For other aspects of the person's behaviour, it may be more appropriate to measure how long an experience lasted, that is, a panic attack (duration). By involving the person in their own assessment, it gives them a sense of responsibility and usefulness. It can empower them to be active participants in their care rather than passive recipients and can help them to gain further insight and understanding of their experiences. This in turn helps them to reframe their sense of self as they begin to recognise strengths they perhaps were unaware of. Recovery-focused self-assessment involves a power shift from professionals to the people they serve, valuing their perspective on their situation and what works for them, supporting informed decision making and assisting them to see their strengths and potential for living.

Logs, diaries and records

Another method useful to empower the person and engage them in the collaborative process of assessment is to encourage them to keep a diary. A diary or log can record a person's daily activities and any related thoughts or emotions. The format of the log can be arranged to suit the person's preference for structured or unstructured formats. It should be agreed and the rationale discussed and how to enter information. An example of a simple cognitive diary can be seen in Table 4.1.

Interviewing/collaborative dialogue

An interview is the most common and most effective way to gain information and an overall assessment of the person. Not only can an interview gain information from questioning but also from observing the person's nonverbal responses and their interaction with the interviewer. An interview is a two-way process in which each person has a specific role, the person is there to explore their experiences and the MHP to facilitate the person's story telling.

Table 4.1   An example of a cognitive diary.

Day	Activity	Thought	Emotion
Monday	Going to the shop for milk	People are looking at me	Become anxious
Tuesday	Talking to a friend	She thinks I am mad	Afraid and embarrassed

An alternative term for this may be collaborative dialogue as interviewing suggests a power differential in which the interviewer has the power and directs the questions, and so as MHPs, it is our responsibility to ensure that a more equal and exploratory approach is used. It is also about 'credulous listening' in believing what is being communicated (Feltham & Dryden, 1993:105). This is particularly important when listening to someone whose sense of perception is altered. It can be difficult to accept what the person is saying, but it is essential that any judgements are withheld. Most would consider that they are good listeners but this is not the case. Many people and practitioners fail to listen, that is, *really* listen to what is being said. When this happens, then people can feel undervalued, judged and even worse worthless; as MHPs, we can prevent this from happening by giving our full attention and actively listening to the person and their story.

Interviews can be structured or unstructured; an unstructured or reflective/collaborative approach is more likely to yield richer, more meaningful information as it is gathered in a less systematic way; rather, it is done in an empathic and intuitive way (Trevithick, 2005). This approach is usually preferable if promoting a recovery-focused assessment as it gives the person the responsibility of identifying their hopes, beliefs, feelings and strengths rather than focusing more on problems or deficits. However, it may be intimidating or overwhelming to have such little structure, and some people may feel they need more prompting from the MHP; this is when a semistructured interview may be more appropriate. A one-size approach does not fit all when striving to promote recovery and it is only by working with the person as a unique individual respecting their vulnerabilities and strengths that we can agree with them and their preferences.

A semistructured interview can be useful as it has certain key areas that the practitioner would use as prompts for the person to respond to, thereby reducing any pressure they may feel to identify areas for discussion.

Formulation
Formulation is a relatively new addition to any care planning process and it originates from psychological theory. However, we can see from the following explanation that it fits with a recovery-focused approach when used in a collaborative way. Bellack and Hensen (1998) state that 'a formulation is designed precisely to fit the individual and is intended to help therapists to derive theoretically based hypotheses about factors that contribute to causing and maintaining their specific problems' (p. 4). A formulation is created with the information gained from the person, and its accuracy and validity should be confirmed with the person so that they have an ownership of it. A formulation then is preferential to diagnosis as it offers a hypothetical framework for interventions that may produce change or benefits for the client. It is within the formulation process that the concepts of recovery and evidence-based approaches can be drawn together to ensure that a shared explanation of the

person's experiences is agreed, and the potential/desirable interventions are identified and selected. Formulation is not just about signs and symptoms but involves arriving at a useful understanding of the person's experiences that is meaningful to them; this is termed the treatment utility (Hayes *et al.*, 1987).

Policy and organisation of care

Assessment within adult mental health services has become an integral part of the care coordination framework (DoH, 1999). Care coordination was introduced in April 2001 following a review of the Care Programme Approach (CPA; DoH, 1990) and the incorporation of Care Management (DoH, 1991) systems that had been established in the early 1990s (DoH, 1993). Care coordination, which incorporates the CPA (DoH, 2006a), is a way of coordinating community health services for people with mental health problems.

The CPA has become an accepted part of practice, despite the continuing lack of strong direct evidence of its value or morality (Sapey, 2004; Kingdon & Amanullah, 2005). Guidance from the Department of Health has refined the original requirements and now specifies that care plans include provision, as necessary, for risk assessment and management, employment, leisure, accommodation and plans to meet carers' needs (DoH, 2006b).

Integrated services, a central requirement of current government thinking, can often be hard to achieve in ways that are respectful and meaningful to service users (Parker, 2001) especially when they employ methods that are bureaucratic, procedurally complex or repetitive (Commission for Social Care Inspection, 2006). Trevithick (2005), drawing on Coulshed and Orme (1998), suggests that assessment should be collaborative (between practitioners, service users and carers) and should incorporate social and environmental factors. Trevithick goes on to add that assessments, whether they are referred to as 'one-off events or ongoing processes, are likely to be similar in practice as 'most acknowledge the importance of monitoring events, updating information and responding to new developments' (Trevithick, 2005:127).

Ixer (2000) points out that both students and experienced workers need opportunities to reflect and develop in order that they might rethink bias and subjectivity. Health and social work practitioners should also attend to more theoretically and personally reflective methodologies if their work is to be truly meaningful, relevant and inclusive (Fook, 2001; Cox & Hardwick, 2002). It is suggested (Trotter & Leech, 2003) that what is often missing from health care practice is a theoretical perspective or what Fook (2002) refers to as critical reflection. Fook argues that this is essential for contextually relevant practice because 'it constitutes an alternative approach to our understanding of knowledge and knowledge creation' (p. 157). Fook advocates that students and practitioners should develop theory from their own experience and, like she has done, learn to bend formal theories to fit their own context, for their own use. Others have worked in this way to develop theoretical and practice models as mechanisms or aide-memoirs to assist them more readily in practice. According to Cutting (1997), models can help practitioners by suggesting:

- Reasons for observed behaviours;
- Therapeutic treatment strategies;
- Role enactment for service user and practitioner.

There are a prolific number of models and theories that can be employed to shape the assessment process and the subsequent care delivery for people experiencing mental health problems. Traditionally, practitioners have been directed to the use of evidence-based models; models that have been subject to systematic review and have been shown to be effective. There has more recently been a move to more recovery-orientated models such as the Wellness Recovery Action Plan (WRAP; Copeland, 2001), Tidal Model (Barker & Buchanan-Barker, 1999; Barker, 2000), Strengths Model (Rapp & Goscha, 2006) and Solution-Focused Model (Berg & De Shazer, 1993). These models are only briefly referred to here.

Wellness recovery action plan
This model was developed by people dealing with mental health problems. It is essentially a guide to self-management and recovery, and it was designed to:

- Decrease and prevent intrusive or troubling feelings and behaviours;
- Increase personal empowerment;
- Improve quality of life;
- Assist people in achieving their own life goals and dreams.

(Copeland, 2001)

Copeland (2001) has shared the model with many people, and she believes that it can be adapted to many other illnesses. The person is given responsibility for developing their own WRAP but they may choose relatives, friends or MHP s to help them.

Tidal Model
This is one of the most well-known models for promoting recovery with projects established in many countries and was developed in the late-1990s in the UK by Barker (2000). It focuses on enabling people to tell their stories, so that they can begin to make sense and derive some meaning from them. The Tidal Model helps people to reclaim their lives as detailed by professionals, which Barker believes is the first step to recovery (Barker & Buchanan-Barker, 1999; Barker, 2000).

Strengths model
At the core of this model is 'a deep belief in the necessity of democracy and the contingent capacity for people to participate in the decisions and actions that define their world' (Saleebey, 1992:8). It has the opposite approach to

most evidence-based models, which tend to identify problems or deficits; instead, it values people's strengths and abilities, hopes and aspirations.

It has several underpinning assumptions:

- Respecting the person's strengths: all people have strengths that they can mobilise to make their lives better;
- Motivation to change is enhanced by building on and acknowledging strengths;
- Cooperation is essential and is a process of exploring strengths;
- Focusing on strengths focuses the work on survival and how this can be achieved;
- The client in their environment is the key to change as the environment contains the resources.

The Strengths Model also underpins the solution-focused model approach, which is also core to the Tidal Model. All have at the core an unconditional valuing of the person experiencing mental health problems, and all believe that it is the person themselves who possesses the resources and abilities to shape their own lives and recover what they can from their experiences.

Practical strategies for promoting recovery-focused assessment
The assessment of an individual with a serious mental illness presents a huge challenge (Gournay, 1996) but has become a major aspect of effective clinical practice (DoH, 1999). Gathering relevant information by selecting the correct process and tools (Gamble & Brennan, 2000) is crucial to understanding the nature of people's experiences and their life.

Preparation for the assessment interview
Preparation and planning are important prior to the interview, whether the person is in a community or a hospital setting as this is often the initial contact with the person and influences the future development of a working relationship. There may be more arranged distractions (Kadushin, 1990) in the home environment that can interfere with the engagement process (a television turned on playing loudly, children playing in the room). The MHP needs to balance the importance of such distractions against empowering the person to be in control of the situation. It would be fine to ask the person if they would mind turning down the TV or asking the children to play in another room, as this would involve a person in the decision-making process; however, the practitioner would then need to respect whatever decision was made.

Other potentially empowering considerations can be:

- Where and when the assessment interview will take place;
- Who may be present other than the practitioner (student nurse, social worker or other colleagues);
- People who the person would like present (friend, carer or advocate);

- How long the interview may last;
- What issues are likely to be covered;
- What, if any, notes will be made or shared and whether they will be recorded during the interview or not.

These can all be discussed at the initial contact so that the person is shown respect and given responsibility in the care planning process. It may be that the person is too unwell in which case the practitioner can consult with the person's carer or advocate who may know of the person's preferences.

The interview
The environment needs to be arranged to promote a physically and psychologically safe feeling for the person, wherever the interview is being held. If in an unfamiliar setting, the person should be reassured regarding privacy and that there will be no interruptions.

Greeting the person and whoever is accompanying them is a way of establishing rapport and demonstrating respect for each individual and also introducing yourself and saying a little about where you work and your role. Also give the person the opportunity to ask any questions from the start, check out their understanding of what will be happening so that they feel as much in control as possible. Another way to initiate the conversation and help the person feel at ease is with small talk: a social chat about their house, how they travelled here or the weather. Any noncontroversial topic is suitable and while this social chat should not continue throughout the interview, it can serve as an icebreaker and allows the person to adapt to the situation, but can become counterproductive if dragged out too long.

The person should then be asked what their priorities or expectations are regarding the meeting, and the MHP should acknowledge whether or not they can be addressed or if there are any other alternatives that may be useful but allowing the person the final decision. Anyone accompanying the person (friend, relative or advocate) should be acknowledged and their needs identified; also their role within the interview should be agreed.

Relationship development
It is essential to demonstrate the following skills in relationship development, during the interview:

- Demonstrating a concern for the issues of the service user and their self-determination;
- Showing an interest, conveying warmth, generating an atmosphere of trust;
- Demonstrating a respect for the service user's individuality;
- Conveying an acceptance of the individual;
- Demonstrating an empathic understanding;

- Conveying a sense of genuineness and authenticity;
- Drawing boundaries on information that may need to be disclosed as necessary and agreeing what may be shared and with whom (Kadushin, 1990).

Explain the role of the interview and its likely format, encourage the use of an unstructured approach initially although this may need to be changed if the person is struggling to tell their story. Intuition will play a large part in that the practitioner should observe for nonverbal cues and respond or adapt their approach accordingly. An opening, inviting question may be sufficient to begin the process followed by occasional encouragement, or more specific questions may be appropriate at times.

Once you have completed the assessment, ensure that you review any notes you have taken with the service user and be prepared to make changes or additions at the user's or advocate's request. Watch your language! Avoid jargon as much as possible and use language that makes the service user an active partner in the planning process rather than the passive recipient of professional decisions. Arrange for the fully written-up assessment to be countersigned by the service user and, if appropriate, the carer.

Preparation for ending should begin at the start of the interview, so that the person is prepared for and expecting the ending. Kadushin (1990) suggests that 'preparation for termination of the interview begins at the very beginning of the interview' (p. 206). An appropriate ending would be to ask what the person feels has been achieved and what they are able to take away with them that is useful. If there are any unresolved issues, then these should be acknowledged and, where appropriate, highlighted as priorities for the next meeting.

Conclusion

In this chapter, we have tried to explore the complex and huge area of assessment. The nature of assessment has been discussed in terms of what it is and how it may be experienced by service users as quite clinical and destructive and how it is more appropriate to consider it as an opportunity for the person to tell their story.

However, at policy and organisational levels, we can witness a history of medical-focused discourse and a current discourse of evidence-based assessment. It has been argued that the recent developments of objective, accurate and scientific procedures in nursing and social work are part of the historical context of modernist empiricism (Iverson *et al.*, 2005). MHPs are caught in a dichotomy between the policy, organisational demands and the needs and aspirations of people. If MHPs are to promote recovery, then the challenge is to let the person define what their recovery is and to collaboratively plan on how that can be achieved. While constrained to some degree with policy guidance, practitioners can minimise the extent of how much of this restricts the person in achieving their recovery. The assessment methods and process can all influence the person's experience, and so practitioners need to choose wisely how assessment is carried out and documented. Subtle changes in practice can lead to a more collaborative approach to assessment and care planning.

All the recovery-focused models offer systems for promoting recovery. However, as already alluded to, recovery should not be another model that becomes professionalised, but one that ensures that people are respected and is implemented according to individual's need. Evidence-based models continue to contribute to improvements in mental health practice but perhaps they should be underpinned with the recovery principles – however, we acknowledge that we have a long distance to travel!

References

American Psychological Association (APA) (2007) *Dictionary.com Unabridged (v 1.1)* [Online]. Available at http://dictionary.reference.com/browse/assess. Accessed on April 2, 2007.

Barker, P.J. (1997) *Assessment in Psychiatric and Mental Health Nursing: In Search of the Whole Person*. Stanley Thornes, Cheltenham.

Barker, P.J. (2000) *The Tidal Model: From Theory to Practice*, University of Newcastle, Newcastle.

Barker, P.J. & Buchanan-Barker, P. (1999) *The Tidal Model: Recovery and Reclamation* [Online]. Available at http://www.tidal-model.com/Recovery.htm. Accessed on May 27, 2013.

Bellack, A.S. & Hensen, M. (1998) *Comprehensive Psychology*. Pergamon Press, New York.

Berg, I.K. & de Shazer, S. (1993) Making numbers talk: language in therapy. In: *New Language of Change* (ed. S. Friedman). Guilford Press, New York.

Commission for Social Care Inspection (2006) *Key Lines of Regulatory Assessment (KLORA): Adult Placement Schemes* [Online]. Available at http://www.csci.org.uk/Docs/klora_aps_080606.doc. Accessed on April 26, 2006.

Copeland, M.E. (2001) Wellness recovery action plan: a system for monitoring, reducing and eliminating uncomfortable or dangerous psychical symptoms and emotional feelings. *Occupational Therapy in Mental Health*, **17** (3/4), 5–21.

Coulshed, V. & Orme, J. (1998) *Social Work Practice: An Introduction*. Macmillan/BASW, Basingstoke.

Cox, P. & Hardwick, L. (2002) Research and critical theory: their contribution to social work education and practice. *Social Work Education*, **21** (1), 35–47.

Cutting, P. (1997) Concepts, models and theories in psychiatric and mental health nursing. In: *Stuart and Sundeen's, Mental Health Nursing, Principles and Practice UK Version* (eds B. Thomas, S. Hardy & P. Cutting). pp. 19–32. Mosby, London.

Deegan, P.E. (1988) Recovery: the lived experience of rehabilitation. *Psychiatric Rehabilitation Journal*, **11**, 11–19.

Department of Health (DoH) (1990) *The Care Programme Approach for People with a Mental Illness Referred to the Special Psychiatric Services*, Joint Health/Social Services Circular, HC (90) 23/LASS (90) 11. HMSO, London.

Department of Health (1991) *Social Services Inspectorate: Care Management and Assessment Guidance*. HMSO, London.

Department of Health (1993) *Services for Mentally Disordered People*, LAC93/10. HMSO, London.

Department of Health (1999) *Effective Care Coordination in Mental Health Services: Modernising the Care Programme Approach, A Policy Booklet*. The Stationery Office, London.

Department of Health (2000) *Framework for the Assessment of Children in Need and their Families*. The Stationery Office, London.

Department of Health (2006a) *Community Care Assessments and Plans*. The Stationery Office, London.

Department of Health (2006b) *Common Assessment Framework* [Online]. Available at http://www.official-documents.gov.uk/document/cm67/6737/6737.pdf. Accessed on May 27, 2013.

Feltham, C. & Dryden, W. (1993) *Dictionary of Counselling*. Whurr Publishers, London.

Fook, J. (2001) Identifying expert social work: qualitative practitioner research. In: *Qualitative Research in Social Work* (eds I. Shaw, & N. Gould). Sage, London.

Fook, J. (2002) *Social Work: Critical Theory and Practice*. Sage, London.

Gamble, C. & Brennan, G. (eds) (2000) *Working With Serious Mental Illness A Manual For Clinical Practice*. Balliere Tindall & RCN, London.

Gournay, K. (1996) Schizophrenia: A review of the contemporary literature and implication for mental health nursing: theory, practice and education. *Journal of Psychiatric and Mental Health Nursing*, **3** (1), 7–12.

Hayes, D. (2005) Social work with asylum seekers and others subject to immigration control. In: *Social Work Futures: Crossing Boundaries, Transforming Practice* (eds R. Adams, L. Dominelli & M. Payne). pp. 182–194. Palgrave Macmillan, Basingstoke.

Hayes, S.C., Nelson, R.O. & Jarrett, R.B. (1987) The treatment utility of assessment: a functional approach to evaluating assessment quality. *American Psychologist*, **42**, 963–974.

Iverson, R.R., Gergen, K.J. & Fairbanks, R.P. (2005) Assessment and social construction: conflict or co-creation? *British Journal of Social Work*, **35** (5), 689–708.

Ixer, G. (2000) Assessing reflective practice: new research findings. *Journal of Practice Teaching*, **2** (3), 19–27.

Kadushin, A. (1990) *The Social Work Interview*, 3rd edn. Columbia University Press, New York.

Kingdon, D.G. & Amanullah, S. (2005) Care programme approach: relapsing or recovering? Making care programming work. *Advances in Psychiatric Treatment*, **11**, 325–329.

Krawiecka, M., Goldberg, D. & Vaughn, M. (1977) A standardised psychiatric assessment scale for rating chronic psychotic patients. *Acta Psychiatrica Scandinavica*, **55**, 299–308.

Lindow, V. (1996) What we want from community psychiatric nurses. In: *Speaking Our Minds* (eds J. Reid, & J. Reynolds). pp. 186–190. Open University Press, Milton Keynes.

O'Sullivan, T. (1999) *Decision Making in Social Work*. Macmillan, Basingstoke.

Parker, J. (2001) Integrating person-centred dementia care in social work and social case practice. *Journal of Social Work*, **1** (3), 329–345.

Priebe, S., Huxley, P., Knight, S., *et al.* (1999) Application and results of the Manchester Short Assessment of Quality of Life. *International Journal of Social Psychiatry*, **45**, 7–12.

Rapp, C.A. & Goscha R.J. (2006) *The Strengths Model: Case Management with People with Psychiatric Disabilities*. Oxford University Press, Oxford.

Repper, J. & Perkins, R. (2003) *Social Inclusion and Recovery: A Model for Mental Health Practice*. Baillière Tindall, Edinburgh.

Saleebey, D. (1992) *The Strengths Perspective in Social Work Practice*. Longman, New York.

Sapey, B. (2004) Practice for what? The use of evidence in social work with disabled people. In: *Social Work and Evidence-Based Practice* (ed. D. Smith). pp. 143–160. Jessica Kingsley Publishers, London.

Trevithick, P. (2005) *Social Work Skills: A Practice Handbook*. Open University Press, Maidenhead.

Trotter, J. & Leech, N. (2003) Linking research, theory and practice in personal and professional development: gender and sexuality issues in social work education. *Social Work Education*, **22** (2), 204–214.

Watkins, P. (2001) *Mental Health Nursing: The Art of Compassionate Care*. Butterworth-Heinemann, London.

Chapter 5

Parity of Esteem

Mike Wren[1] and Natalie Iley[2]

[1]Teesside University, UK
[2]Stockton Borough Council, UK

For Sheila (23.8.35 – 27.10.12) and Madge

> *The best and most beautiful things cannot be seen or even touched they must be felt with the heart*
>
> —Helen Keller

Introduction

Our chapter aims to illustrate the importance of consolidating the core concepts, potential impact and practical application of essential lifestyle-planning experiences, as derived from the person experiencing mental distress and those closest to them. It will also highlight what will be referred to as a series of 'parity of esteem considerations' that we believe are essential to enhancing the future of mental, emotional, social and physical wellbeing of a person experiencing mental distress, while striving to establish how the deployment of preventative, person-centred perspectives can promote life choice opportunities that strive to personalise rather than pathologise the lifestyle of a person and those closest to them. This proactive response equally celebrates the valiant contributions of people experiencing mental distress and those closest to them, and their bid to achieve the ultimate goal of reciprocating a genuine sense of parity of esteem captured in unison with many other people in society.

This chapter will further seek to develop understanding of our chosen parity of esteem considerations, based upon the 'lived experience' perspective of the person experiencing mental distress and acknowledging (for some) the crucial involvement of those closest to them. This is done by further

Care Planning in Mental Health: Promoting Recovery, Second Edition.
Edited by Angela Hall, Michael Wren and Stephan D. Kirby.
© 2013 John Wiley & Sons, Ltd. Published 2013 by John Wiley & Sons, Ltd.

contrasting coherent personal aspirations to both combine and contemporise, a series of collegiate, person centred and recovery orientated principles into a practicable reality. These principles realistically strive to identify with our series of parity of esteem considerations and are capable of enhancing the person's reclamation of their 'own' sense of recovery of interdependent functioning and to establish an identity within a meaningful lifestyle. Such an identity is weighted alongside comparable features of essential lifestyle planning and is aimed at moving the rhetorical debate onto a more meaningful, purposeful reality. We must constantly acknowledge that the collective 'passionate petitioning' of the person experiencing mental distress, those closest to them and their community allies, must always be at the forefront of all our collective endeavours, in order to succeed in proactively promoting recovery of interdependent functioning (Hall & Wren, 2008).

Parity of esteem considerations

Our response to 'How different would services look if their primary focus was to enable people to use and develop their skills, make the most of their assets, and pursue their aspirations' (Repper & Perkins, 2003:11) is to acknowledge from the outset the importance and urgency of developing a future collective of 'recovery brokers' whose primary focus is to proactively promote the recovery of interdependent functioning by consistently cocreating with the person (incremental) step changes needed to unravel the professional orientation (model focus) to the active promotion of the person and their individually constructed narrative towards a more holistic (person-centred focus). Recovery brokers also contribute considerably to the cofacilitation of creative interactions between the person's natural ability to forge emotional resilience from within turbulent or adverse events as a direct result of tapping into their own, often unseen, reserves of 'social, mental and recovery capital' (Kanter, 1994; Sainsbury Centre for Mental Health, 2001; SCIE, 2004; DoH, 2010).

Essential to achieving such personal self-fulfilment requires a concerted renewal of a relationship-based perspective, to build elements of sustainable considerations to translate into humane resource capabilities to focus, plan, and achieve. With each capability being translated via the person experiencing mental distress, as well as the mutual efforts of self and others, we all bid to define, or maybe redefine, a unique story that rejuvenates hope for a better lifestyle and the achievement of life chance opportunities for the person and not forgetting those closest to them. Thus challenging preoccupations with averting, rather than enabling, or moreover sharing, risks that are often perceived to be wholly created from the varying causes of a person's mental distress. The further championing of person-focused parity of esteem considerations, and their actual interpretation, needs to be explored from a uniquely individual perspective too. We need to continually strive, alongside the person experiencing mental distress, those closest to them and their community of allies, to uphold the credentials of our collective of recovery brokers who each endorse collegiate acceptance and by doing so, we will do our very best to serve people on their unique journey towards promoting interdependent recovery through effectively 'communicating', 'collaborating' and 'coordinating' our efforts to restore their hopes, aspirations and deliberations to establish the person's real lifestyle choices. Equally, these clusters of interlinking parity of esteem considerations are directly related to some basic, yet fundamental, tenets that allow parallels to be drawn between human rights, resources and responsibilities to assist with embedding an incremental shift towards a culture or mind-set, that is open to evolving the future development of a collaborative of recovery brokers, in context and with due regard to three core themes namely: People, Potential and Places.

People

Striving to listen, respond, engage and mobilise involvement on the basis of creatively empowering people, to identify the realistic changes they *want* to make to their lifestyle opportunities, choices and chances.

Potential

Arriving at a cocreated understanding of the person, their support networks, and their relationship to community-orientated opportunities, to fulfil in some measure a meaningful lifestyle. By negotiating with community allies and converting community resources to build capacity to meet specific aspects of the person's narrative, their individual biography of their lifestyle. Further, the cocreation of costings based on entitlement, contributions, and considerations as captured within person-centred plans and, thereby, identifying fairer, innovative, moral and transparent legal methods to obtain aspects of funding. These contribute to the avoidance (wherever possible) of hospitalisation or rehospitalisation, while promoting recovery by initiating a lifestyle plan, that releases the person's reserves of recovery capital. Ultimately, ensuring that all of our personal interactions are strengthened by coherent, citizen-focused values, shared capabilities, accountabilities and positive due regard for the person, where national policy seeks to address the responsibility for the support and appropriate person-focused regulation of a local collaborative of recovery brokers.

Places

To cocreate opportunities for interacting with people experiencing mental distress via peer support, and user-led community groups acknowledging, and indeed further encouraging, the active input of family members, friends and a variety of other community allies. By collectively creating a forum, where we can together appropriately challenge prescriptive or discriminatory inhibitors, we can achieve positive life chance outcomes, in order to really deliver personalised experiences, from within existing opportunities, or naturally occurring events evolving from within localised community resources.

Essentially, this involves moving alongside the person experiencing mental distress and those closest to them, with a real sense of natural empathy and entering into the person's subjective world to feel what it might be like for people experiencing mental distress and discover what he or she may be thinking and then conveying that understanding back to them. Instead of overtly pathologising, we should instead strive to enable the person to reach their true potential to effect change capable of proactively promoting recovery. Keeping in touch with self is equally important in relation to conveying natural empathy, for the capacity to be in touch with the person experiencing mental distress, or those closest to them, is largely related to our capacity and ability to acknowledge 'our own' life experiences. Before we can understand the power of emotion in the life of the person experiencing mental distress or those closest to them, it is necessary to discover its importance from their and our own terms of reference (SCIE, 2004).

Empowering others has created an explosion of interest especially towards cultivating the idea of empowerment transcending across the helping professions. This is further reflected in broader parity of esteem considerations within mental health and the active promotion of recovery, in that it transcends conventional politics and ideologies by seeking to address both the personal and political by uniting the two. It is now a central pillar in political, social policy, educational, cultural, sexual, personal and managerial discourses as well as entering popular usage and policy debates. However, we must remain mindful that concern still remains from groups representing the person with the mental health problems and carer groups and that these ideas or considerations do not become reduced to an overly jargon-laden use of terms of reference and thereby lack clarity for the individual who is experiencing mental distress, those closest to them and their community allies (SCIE, 2004).

In the fascinating interchange of striving to empower people experiencing mental distress and those closest to them to pursue the active promotion of recovery due regard to the parity of esteem considerations (suggested here) are reliant on the creation of a real sense of union between discharging power toward the person, that aims to make meaningful changes in their lives, against an ever changing socio-economic landscape and for some diminishing life chance opportunities in response to an extremely adverse economic and social capital reinvestment environments. However, such humane responses towards enabling individuals, families, groups and communities to increase their personal, interpersonal, socio-economic and political strength and influence towards improving their own life chance opportunities are, therefore, the hallmarks of real empowering practice as measured by the person, their lifestyle and future lived outcomes alongside their chosen community allies (Warren, 2007; McLaughlin, 2009).

Outcomes which often need to be tempered (for some people) against the initial societal perceptions of the person at the height of their mental distress, which can often include feelings of mistrust, arrogance, aggression, or contempt from others towards them and vice versa, and where such feelings can often occupy and resonate throughout your, or our whole, psyche too, and at the very point of feeling at your or our most distressed, vulnerable and fearful.

Perhaps we should be persuaded then, that our parity of esteem considerations should begin with an open acknowledgement that our fixations, insights and habits are for the most part shared characteristics, and that professionals alone should not have the boldness, insight and open mindedness to expose and name the causes of a person's mental distress. Rather, there is a need to collaborate with their personal capital and capabilities, rather than colluding with those life chance opportunity-inhibiting labels, that far too often stereotype people experiencing mental distress as being radically different to others (Saleebey, 2009; Fry, 2010).

Personalising parity of esteem

To understand the personalising of parity of esteem, we have to understand distress, confusion and pain experienced by people with mental health problems without becoming confused, distressed or in pain ourselves, and most especially within their presence (Biesteck, 1961; SCIE, 2004). By contrasting this mutual acknowledgment of human frailty and vulnerability alongside inner strength and personal resilience, or what Saleebey (2009) refers to as 'survivor's pride', is the resounding need to personalise our own mask of security, ease, self-confidence and reassurance that at times we all wear, and which all too often betrays the real conditions of anxiety, self-doubt, disgust and fear that often lingers beneath the surface (Fry, 2010). The person's sense of physical as well as mental wellbeing opportunities and their link to essential lifestyle planning cannot therefore be underestimated when striving to sustain a livelihood, family life, leisure time and essentially their status of citizen. This is especially so as they embark on their own journey of actively striving to pursue finding hope from personal adversity on the basis of recovery. This is a journey that is built upon their reservoir of human resources of inner strength and resilience to stimulate those personalised life choice opportunities being made available within society. It is underpinned by a series of compatible parity of esteem considerations by engaging with people, then matching their potential *to* opportunities available within places that could actually contribute to realising ambitions or the fulfilment of aspirations.

Such reciprocal experiences chart the real-life accounts and insights that have influenced the many political, societal, medical and social developments in the active promotion of recovery. This is particularly true when we begin the journey by personalising these lived experiences, not just as concepts to inform a series of parity of esteem considerations but to stimulate practical and achievable realities for the person experiencing mental distress and those people closest to them. This journey, it is acknowledged from the outset, transcends many differing thresholds from human pain to self-pride and the eventual realisation of the person's true potential.

Where these features of humane existence are equally characterised by the lived experiences of many people trying to make sense of, and cope with, such mental distress, in all of its varying guises. With each threshold confronted on a daily basis, like a personalised passport stamped on a unique journey of expressing the realisation of the person's own narrative of recovery, essentially trying to salvage for them, a realistic sense of a parity of esteem that equates to feeling genuinely valued as a person, alongside their families, friends and community allies as contributory members of localised communities.

Personal narrative accounts chronicle the emergent themes which suggest that the emergence of recovery brokers should continue their preventative pursuit of securing social justice for all, in the name of achieving some person-focused balances between competing legal parameters, alongside some extremely complex as well as conflicting versus consensual issues, in particular, those experiences or opportunities that contribute to either the person's recovery or relapse, namely: employment, housing, education, finances, family relationships. Also, acting as both challenges and opportunities, in response to the recurring dilemmas of, should we detain (on behalf of society) using the law or seek voluntary participation or community-based action?

This is perhaps the critical part of personalising the recovery journey, as we each carefully steer a humanistic course of meandering between the morality of protecting the rights of a citizen experiencing mental distress, alongside exploring preventative opportunities to minimise admission or detention in hospital and above all else to minimise the risk of the potential for harm towards themselves or the wider public. Although this is a highly emotive interchange, it can also provide the crossroads for our own self-reflection too. By preparing ourselves to challenge, and be challenged by, the very perceptions of the person at the heights of their mental distress we, the perceived powerful professionals, need to juggle with the fact that on the one hand, we are determining whether to remove someone's liberty, while on the other, encouraging voluntary actions and proactive outcomes as societal agents of social control and arriving at a consensus to avoid (wherever possible) the need for hospitalisation or rehospitalisation.

We could, while working together across boundaries of indifference or territorialism, strive to establish approaches that encourage notions of involvement rather than the punitive connotation of silo-focused interventions. We can all share and combine our compatible spheres of recovery brokerage based primarily upon transferable and portable knowledge, skills and experiential insights, as gleaned from the person experiencing mental distress, which also includes capturing the essential insights of those closest to them and add this to our own motivation for facilitating person-centred, recovery-focused outcomes. This will result in us offering the person whose life it is a real sense of parity of esteem, in relation to the life changing decisions made with, and ultimately alongside, them, as well as those most close to them, who are also travelling on this journey of unpredictable feelings, thoughts and actions towards proactively promoting the recovery of interdependent functioning.

For people experiencing mental distress to achieve some realistic life chance opportunities, the commonality of human conditions need to be considered in context with ensuring that the mutual exploration of parity of esteem considerations is further encouraged to ensure that they can coexist between everyone involved from the very outset of involvement. This is achieved by engaging with the person, regardless of their reason for involvement, position or status and based on their skilful ability to appropriately delegate (wherever possible) any domains of potential power perceived or otherwise (Fook, 2002).

Each person, and their actions, involved, is capable of being judged against a comparable set of 'citizen focused' values and principles, particularly when considering the provision of positive life choice opportunities essential to the person and their lifestyle. For they transcend the challenges and opportunities emerging from the smouldering embers of experiencing relapse, onwards to the ultimate goal of recovery, or vice versa, and as experienced by working alongside such intelligent, unique, creative and capable people.

However, before we can all begin to congratulate ourselves on being the spokesperson for humanity (Fry, 2010), we need to remind ourselves that we can only collectively claim this accolade, when we have really tried all options available to us to capture the narrative of the person directly experiencing, or who has experienced, such extremes of mental distress along the road between relapse and recovery, namely their families, carers or other community allies. This is another essential consideration, as we strive to really ascertain what the collective vision of what recovery actually means to the person and more importantly for them. We then galvanise together our mutual interpretations to reflect, as well as reciprocate, our collective understanding and knowledge(s) to facilitate a series of realistic, achievable and practicable life chance opportunities to incrementally emerge.

Exploring these themes together is also an attempt to engage with the self-discovery of ourselves and others who are each actively pursuing the reclamation of self-respect, identity and proactive promotion of their mental, physical and social wellbeing. To work alongside families or carers, and within collaborative communities, could create some fascinating environments for such powerful interrelationships to be developed. We all then travel along this path of least resistance, spurring us into action via our collective endeavours to promote recovery. The concept of promoting recovery by utilising a person-centred and parity esteem focus is not unique, nor is it quantifiably straightforward or exact. In fact, it is contested and contestable, which also provides the stimulus for us to consider how we can pursue it even further.

The fact that this dual focus is so diverse, makes it all the more relevant and contemporary where it is also founded upon an informed view of proactive engagement of people experiencing mental distress and those closest to them (Repper & Perkins, 2003; Hall *et al.*, 2008). This can also create further opportunities for the catalysts of uniqueness, creativity, originality and diversity to come together, for just as with colour, or sense and pain, we can never know whether any of our experiences, perceptions or sensations of recovery is the same as others (Fry, 2010). However, our own sense of self-discovery and further understanding of a recovery-focused personal narrative, as derived from actual lived experiences, are preferred here. Especially when they are balanced more evenly against a wholly professional body regulated, central Government target-driven model, which prompts us to restate the urgent need to place a relationship-based perspective at the heart of regulation, rather than the other way around (Ruch *et al.*, 2010).

To measure the success of relationship-based perspectives, relies upon charting life chance outcomes with the person, which are not overly reliant upon prescriptive monitoring which can merely serve to justify and maintain a beleaguered and overly bureaucratic process within a system that is centrally controlled and which for some people (experiencing mental distress) can prove to be an inaccessible hierarchy. This will require us to continue the building or rebuilding of strong working alliances to truly embrace parity of esteem, not as a philosophical ideal or political notion, but as a radical, practical reality delivered via recovery-focused and person-centred outcomes. The realism confronting us all that no matter how confident we may appear to others, inside, we are all, potentially, sobbing, scared and uncertain for much of the time (Fry, 2010).

Giving consideration to the current climate of a global economic downturn, and with it the potential dawning of a human resource tsunami, one that has the potential to erupt and scatter remnants of lost opportunities, will prevent us demonstrating our combined skills, strengths, inner resources, capacity and emotional resilience to be fully realised. These scatterings of lost opportunities are the very hallmarks for revisiting the scope and potential of social capital, mental or moreover recovery capital (Kanter, 1994; DoH, 2010) to exemplify what is required to achieve some sustainable degree of success in trying to reinvigorate a person's claim to parity of esteem which is inextricably linked to their own identity and purpose in life.

By bringing together people, we can facilitate potentiality via person-centred plans and stimulate those places that can be utilised to foster the notion that we are not alone, as we marvel together at what, for some, may be seen as the unpredictability of the human mind or for others the strangeness of human nature (Fry, 2010). While for others this creates some real potential to increase momentum, refocus lost ambition or regain the pride of promoting recovery as a worthwhile citizen striving to achieve some degree of interdependence by forging a meaningful identity within their local community and wider society. The conjoining of parity of esteem considerations with the proactive promotion of recovery is inextricably linked to us all seeking to personalise the experience of recovery, to change for the better, the experience of using services and the relationship between workers and those whom we serve (Repper & Perkins, 2003).

The collective pursuit of personalising parity of esteem must acknowledge from the outset that human vulnerabilities can often act as the catalyst, in unison with a person experiencing mental distress, to tapping into the reserves of their well of inner strengths, resources and personal resilience. Each aspect has the potential to produce far-reaching consequences, and impacts, for sustaining that person's livelihood, family life, leisure time and essentially their status of citizenship to really pursue finding hope from personal adversity on the basis of recovering their own reservoir of self-belief to succeed. Ultimately, they will develop the ability to function as independently as possible, remembering that none of us are truly independent; rather, we are interdependent on each other for our ultimate survival, existence and fulfilment.

Parity of esteem

From rhetoric to reality

We need to continue to seek to avoid prescriptive frameworks to further translate the realities of personalising recovery alongside the latest proposals from Government that are particularly influenced by policies created primarily from user-led consultative insights. When these (following) themes are taken together with our parity of esteem considerations and personalising recovery perspectives, they can each offer some encouraging responses to strengthen the potential contributions and future development of generic responses, mapped out within a series of holistic essential lifestyle-planning considerations. Enhancing life chance opportunities and outcomes for people experiencing mental distress and those closest to them, in collaboration (wherever possible) with a collective of recovery brokers and community allies galvanising together their combined efforts and collective pursuit of embedding the overarching notions of:

Freedom: By giving people control, their potential for improved mental well-being will increase;

Fairness: By not colluding with the stereotypical labels or stigma and making explicit links with the nine protected characteristics as enshrined within DoH (2010);

Responsibility: By everyone planning together in the cocreation of positive experiences of supportive and enabling recovery-focused opportunities to emerge;

The emergence of the latest national, international and user-led policy initiatives to promote recovery are emphasised in Objective 4, 'Positive Care & Support', and Objective 6, 'Tackling Stigma', within *No Health without Mental Health* (DoH, 2011) and associated parity of esteem considerations. Each aspect acknowledges that people, when planning their individual recovery journey, need to experience positive, personalised support, and be enabled by giving choices, and greater control, to plan their aspirations and accorded respect as individuals. This is based upon their individual stories and their personal narratives which provide the foundations for their support. Positive experiences that have originated from personalised lifestyle planning to assist in building upon social, mental or recovery capital are likely to further encouraged when people experiencing mental distress, those closest to them and their community allies.

Connect with other people: Especially those closest to or around them (family and community);

Remain active: By regular uptake of exercise or activities;

Take notice: Of the world around them to grasp their own sense of potential and opportunities;

Keep learning: New skills, new things and taking on challenges;

Eventually give something back: By volunteering, helping others to help themselves (peer support) to increase participation, raise self-esteem and increase mental wellbeing via determined collective action;

Tackle stereotypical stigma: The Government concedes that this aspect will need more major and sustained social movement and collective action with the potential renaissance for charitable, community and self-help groups emerging with community-based projects that embrace and advocate for meaningful employment, affordable housing and educational opportunities.

Each aspect is firmly enshrined within the DoH (2010) and its clear emphasis of responsibilities on organisations or employers towards those people deemed under the previous Disability Discrimination Act (DoH, 2005) definition as having a physical or mental impairment which has a substantial or long term (i.e., over at least 12 months) adverse effect on their abilities to carry out normal day-to-day activities are also being coherently considered within the nine protected characteristics of the DoH (2010).

Translated into a practical reality, these concepts may not necessarily take mountains of public money, that may or is not readily available anyway, but it will undoubtedly require the efficient use, or the redeployment, of human resources. Also required would be the reestablishing, or reinvigorating, of physical resources, as 'environments of engagement' within local community resources (i.e., leisure centres, voluntary groups, user-led action networks or cooperatives). However, we would advocate that the lessons learnt in previous developments, relating to enabling personalised support, are both recognised and collectively replicated, rather than being rejected or left to become redundant. In order to confront together the challenges that lie ahead, we could celebrate the opportunities to maximise the many physical, mental, emotional and economical benefits to be transcended throughout our many diverse interactions and, where we really aim to further stimulate, via the notion of a 'compassionate regeneration of people' to live within their own communities and by ensuring that our actions are consistently founded upon remaining:

Person centred: Suiting the person and that they fit with their lifestyle aspirations;

Clear: With meaningful outcomes for the person to realistically achieve;

Practical: The person should know how they actually could achieve their desired outcomes;

Safe: The person should make sure they and others are not put at unnecessary risk (Risk Enabling versus Risk Averse). There should be considerations given to safeguarding mental, emotional, financial and physical health wellbeing;

Self determined: The person should be in as much control as is feasibly possible: considerations of empowering versus enhancements;

Managed: Clear lines of management and responsibility for actions, outcomes and opportunities being collectively realised: considerations of Care versus Control;

In budget: Where a personal budget is established as the most appropriate resource to sustain the compassionate regeneration of people and associated activities, it is essential that the person is encouraged not to spend more than has been agreed, and this is based on the underpinning legal and moral principles of the person's capacity. These should include consideration of the differences, legal, logistical and any potential overlaps, with individual Health Budgets, Personal Budgets or whether (section 117) After Care payments could be legitimately utilised in the future financial and political landscape to complement the essential lifestyle-planning considerations, that would add value to the developments envisaged within this chapter. Such personal budgets are underpinned and subsequently delivered by a committed collective of recovery brokers whose primary focus is to assist people to remain living within their own communities and to avoid, wherever possible, the need for hospitalisation or rehospitalisation.

Equally, these financial considerations should be unequivocally underpinned by a much clearer understanding of the respective roles, responsibilities and subsequent recourse to resources being directly applied across professional boundaries as delivered by a collective of recovery brokers. We can then begin to challenge restrictive, distant and silo-thinking approaches to ensure people experiencing mental distress and those closest to them can be encouraged to legitimately pursue their right to an individual budget. One based upon accessibility to flexible funding mapped to a series of transparent, accountability and capacity-focused principles, many of which are already enshrined in (UK) mental health law. This would forge together, as far as is feasibly possible, the future direction of person-centred policy, plans and places, with the ultimate aim of encouraging individual potential.

Any future developments must consult with the past, particularly in relation to stimulating use of health flexibilities (DoH, 1999, 2000, 2001, 2007), and with them, develop a real commitment to pool resources in order to further plan for the future of the interdependency and the abilities of the statutory sector, the voluntary sector and local communities to really forge together with lasting and trusting relationships. Mental health provision will not be transformed on a shoestring, and what must be realised is that although the costs of the required changes may well prove to be significant, these are likely to be far less than the longer term costs associated with piecemeal changes which lead to shattered lives.

Equally by working together with a range of people, in response to a multiplicity of human needs, diverse circumstances and unique aspirations can often be perceived as being easy when things are going well, but it takes time, effort and commitment to stay together during the testing or tough times that will undoubtedly arise too. If the continued modernisation of mental health provision is to have a meaningful and longer term impact on the lives of people experiencing mental distress and those closest to them, then one key deficiency of the current law or policy directives that needs urgent attention is the lack of a coherent person-centred legal framework that specifically promotes recovery and the personalising of life chance opportunities for people experiencing mental distress and specifically for those closest to them. The future delivery of community-orientated, personalised support and enablement, alongside the essential considerations for effectively safeguarding the mental, emotional, physical and financial wellbeing of vulnerable adults, would be improved immeasurably. Such pieces of legislation should be brought together into a consolidating Act in order to address the current arrangements that, despite a plethora of legislation, still remain piecemeal, confusing and not at all user friendly (Sardar, 2004; Glasby, 2006; Johns, 2006).

References

Biesteck, F. (1961) *The Casework Relationship*. Allen & Unwin, London.

Department of Health (DoH) (1999) *Health Act*. DoH, London.

Department of Health (2000) *Care Standards Act*. DoH, London.

Department of Health (2001) *Health & Social Care Act*. DoH, London.

Department of Health (2007) *Putting People First: A Shared Vision and Commitment to the Transformation of Adult Social Care*. DoH, London.

Department of Health (2010) *Equality Act*. DoH, London.

Department of Health (2011) *No Health without Mental Health*. DoH, London.

Fook, J. (2002) *Social Work Critical Theory and Practice*. Sage, London.

Fry, S (2010) *The Fry Chronicles*. Penguin Books, London.

Glasby, J. (2006) Are partnerships worth? Health special. *Community Care Magazine*, **15** (12), 2–33.

Hall, A. & Wren, M. (2008) The context and nature of care planning in mental health. In: *Care Planning in Mental Health: Promoting Recovery* (eds A. Hall, M. Wren & S.D. Kirby). pp. 3–23. Wiley-Blackwell, Oxford.

Hall, A., Wren, M. & Kirby, S. D. (2008) Reflections on the future. In: *Care Planning in Mental Health: Promoting Recovery* (eds A. Hall, M. Wren & S.D. Kirby). pp. 255–262. Wiley-Blackwell, Oxford.

Johns, R. (2006) *Using the Law in Social Work*. Learning Matters, Exeter.

Kanter, R. (1994) *The Change Masters*. Routledge, London.

McLaughlin, H. (2009) *Service User Research in Health and Social Care*. Sage, London.

Repper, J. & Perkins, R. (2003) *Social Inclusion and Recovery: A Model for Mental Health*. Bailliere Tindall, Edinburgh.

Ruch, G., Turney, D. & Ward, A. (2010) *Relationship-Based Social Work: Getting to the Heart of Practice*, Jessica Kingsley Publishers, London.

Sainsbury Centre for Mental Health (2001) *Mental Health Policy: The Challenges Facing the Government*, SCMH, London.

Saleebey, D. (2009) *The Strengths Perspective in Social Work Practice*, 4th edn. Allyn & Bacon, Boston.

Sardar, S. (2004) Mental health needs a lifeline. *Community Care Magazine*, **11**(17), 37.

Social Care Institute of Excellence (SCIE) (2004) *Teaching and Learning Communication Skills in Social Work*, SCIE, London.

Warren, J. (2007) *Service User and Carer Participation in Social Work*, Learning Matter, Exeter.

Chapter 6

Holistic Care: Physical Health, Mental Health and Social Factors

Teresa Moore and Scott Godfrey

Teesside University, UK

The term, 'wellbeing' refers to the achievement of a positive physical, social and mental state as opposed to the absence of mental illness or disease (DoH, 2011a). Wellbeing is associated with improved physical health and life expectancy, better educational achievement and employment rates and productivity, reduced antisocial behaviour and criminality and reduced levels of risky behaviours including smoking and alcohol and substance misuse (DoH, 2011a).

However, it is acknowledged that there are certain groups within society who are particularly susceptible to developing chronic/life-threatening illnesses due to a combination of social, environmental and lifestyle factors (DoH, 2011a) and in turn, these people are also identified as high risk for developing mental illness with all its consequences; morbidity and mortality rates are generally higher because of increased exposure to lifestyle risk factors such as smoking, poor diet and sedentary lifestyle (Nash, 2011), and they are at increased risk of suicide (DoH, 2012a). In areas of high unemployment and social deprivation, health inequalities rise proportionately (DoH, 2011a) and subsequently, mental health service users are at a higher risk of developing many physical health conditions than the mentally well population. Those with severe forms of mental illness are at increased risk of physical illness (Brown *et al.*, 2000; Cohen & Hove, 2001), and can expect a lifespan considerably shortened as a direct result of mental illness (Lambert *et al.*, 2003; DoH, 2011b). They are also less likely to access public health initiatives including health screening (Cohen & Hove, 2001), making it less likely they would benefit from early detection of disease. Physical illnesses include higher rates of cardiac and cardiovascular disease, respiratory disease, obesity, cancer and diabetes (Cohen & Hove, 2001; Lambert *et al.*, 2003; BHF, 2012). Additionally, the mentally ill experience more long-term harm from alcohol misuse, illicit substance abuse and smoking (DoH, 2011a).

Care Planning in Mental Health: Promoting Recovery, Second Edition.
Edited by Angela Hall, Michael Wren and Stephan D. Kirby.
© 2013 John Wiley & Sons, Ltd. Published 2013 by John Wiley & Sons, Ltd.

The Department of Health (DoH, 1990) recommended that health services should adopt an holistic approach to the assessment and treatment of mental health service users, and *The National Service Framework (NSF) for Mental Health* (DoH, 1999) made explicit recommendations to support the physical health care of people with mental health problems, acknowledging the contribution made by social deprivation and social exclusion. The concept of holistic nursing assessment and care delivery was further promoted in the *Chief Medical Officer's Review of Nursing* (DoH, 2006a), reinforcing the need for mental health care professionals to develop the required knowledge and skills to assess and care for mental health service users' physical health needs as well as their primary mental health presentation, and though the NMC (2010) states that all registered nurses must have the knowledge and skills required to provide holistic care, and competency frameworks clearly identify the requirement for achievement of physical healthcare skills, this philosophy is not yet embedded in clinical practice. Despite these pledges, it is becoming increasingly apparent that the *needs of all* are not being adequately addressed. Equity and parity of esteem are still elusive objectives, especially for those with mental health-related illness/injury. Despite these statistics, mental illness is often portrayed as the 'poorer relation' to physical health and given lesser priority (AoMRC, 2008). Recent papers such as *No Health without Mental Health* (DoH, 2011b), and the implementation framework which followed (DoH, 2012b), appear to signal a significant change in direction, with the Department of Health striving for 'parity of esteem', requesting organisations to recognise that physical health is no more important than mental health (and vice versa). Service users have expressed the expectation that mental health nurses should provide practical and social support as well as psychological support (Bee *et al.*, 2008).

Recovery

Mental illness is closely associated with social exclusion, and the range of those adversely affected include the unemployed, victims of abuse including domestic violence, the homeless, those with alcohol and substance dependence, black and ethnic minorities and refugees and those incarcerated in prisons. Additionally, children from low-income families and those living with chronic physical illness or disability are also at higher risk of developing mental ill health (DoH, 1999). Maintaining social networks, being part of a community, and staying active all benefit health and wellbeing in later life (DoH, 2011a). The stigma attached to these groups within the population may be the biggest barrier to recovery in mental health (Nash, 2011).

The 2012 strategy, *Compassion in Practice* (DoH, 2012b), identifies the skills required of the nurse, which contribute to successful outcomes for clients/patients. The '6 Cs' encompass the core skills required of the nurse in order to deliver high quality nursing care:

- **Care:** is our core business and that of our organisations and the care we deliver helps the individual person and improves the health of the whole community. Caring defines us and our work. People receiving care expect it to be right for them consistently throughout every stage of their life;
- **Compassion:** is how care is delivered through relationships based on empathy, respect and dignity. It can also be described as intelligent kindness, and is central to how people perceive their care;
- **Competence:** means nurses must be able to understand an individual's health and social needs. Their expertise, clinical and technical knowledge for delivering care and treatment must be based on research and evidence;
- **Communication:** is central to successful caring relationships and team working. Listening is as important as what nurses say and do and essential for 'no decisions about me without me'. Communication is the key to a good workplace with benefits for staff and patients alike;
- **Courage:** enables nurses to do the right thing for the people. It means speaking up when there are concerns and having the personal strength and vision to innovate and embrace new ways of working;
- **Commitment:** A commitment to patients and populations is a cornerstone of what we do. We need to build on our commitment to improve the care and experience of our patients to take action to make this vision and strategy a reality for all and meet the health and social care challenges ahead.

(DoH, 2012b)

Promoting health and recovery

The importance of exercise within the general population is accepted as a means of promoting good physical health, including reducing the risk of heart disease by 30% (BHF, 2012). In recent years, the benefit of exercise for people with mental illness, either as a single therapeutic intervention or as an adjunct to treatment, has been recognised (Crone & Guy, 2008). Exercise is considered to be good for mental health overall. Meaningful activity is associated with general wellbeing, promotes self-esteem, socialisation, with subsequent boost in confidence and consequently contributes to positive mental health (Crone & Guy, 2008). The lack of it, associated with a sedentary lifestyle, is thought to contribute to some mental illnesses (Wand & Murray, 2008). Though the Department of Health (DoH, 2006b) recommends exercise as a therapeutic intervention for mental health service users, its implementation is rarely apparent in mainstream mental health services (Callaghan,

2004). Since mental health service users have a shorter life expectancy than the general population (Cohen & Hove, 2001), health promotion within mental health nursing should be a priority, and exercise would provide the foundation for general health improvement and increased life expectancy. Of course, the difficulty is that many of those experiencing mental illness have reduced levels of motivation; this is compounded by a combination of weight gain caused by increased appetite and lifestyle and the sedative effect of antipsychotic and mood-stabilising drug therapies affecting a person's perception in relation to body image (Johnstone *et al.*, 2009). This double jeopardy results in a low take-up of exercise as part of a healthy lifestyle.

Mental health nurses confirm their commitment to promoting holistic nursing (Brimblecombe *et al.*, 2007), and identify some of the barriers and suggestions for promotion of holistic care. Lack of knowledge and skill of some mental health nurses to the physical health needs of mental health service users affecting their confidence was suggested as one barrier to holistic care (Howard & Gamble, 2011). It is evident that many mental health professionals lack expertise in recognising and nursing clients with physical health needs, including any rapid deterioration in the physical condition of their clients (Brimblecombe *et al.*, 2007). Education and expansion of current physical assessment skills, both at pre- and postregistration, were identified as prerequisites to high-quality nursing; the role of the mental health nurse as health promoter was also identified as key in the development of strategies to address the problems associated with drug and alcohol abuse and smoking. Though many mental health nurses feel more confident about directing their skills towards service users' mental health, those same service users have expressed the desire to learn more about adopting a healthy lifestyle (Verhaeghe *et al.*, 2011). Howard & Gamble (2011) also suggested that there is a lack of acknowledgement by some mental health nurses of the need to diversify from what they perceive to be their primary role, and they consider physical health care to be the responsibility of medics and adult nurses, failing to recognise their responsibility in this vital aspect of care. The following features are seen to be contributory to the core considerations given to the delivery of quality care experiences.

Physical considerations for quality of care

Coronary heart disease is the foremost cause of death in the UK, with a clear correlation between the disease and social circumstances. In 2008, rates were 50% higher in socially deprived areas of the UK, with a marked North/South divide (DoH, 2004; BHF, 2012). In 2010, 65 000 people died of coronary heart disease (BHF, 2012). High-risk factors include many behaviours described as 'lifestyle choices', including poor diet, physical inactivity, smoking and heavy consumption of alcohol (BHF, 2012). Risk for coronary heart disease and cardiovascular disease is increased by consumption of saturated fat which increases cholesterol in the blood resulting in atherosclerosis (BHF, 2012). A healthy diet of fruit, vegetables and protein in balanced measures maintains a healthy cardiovascular system, reducing the risk of stroke (BHF, 2012). Mortality due to cardiac and cardiovascular disease is higher in those with mental illness (Lambert *et al.*, 2003), and reduced life expectancy due to cardiovascular disease is the leading cause of premature death in those with schizophrenia (Ohlsen, 2011), due to the combination of lifestyle factors and psychotropic medication used to control symptoms of mental illness.

Obesity is determined by the measurement of a person's Body Mass Index (BMI), which identifies inappropriate weight for the height and build of an individual. Britain is now the most obese nation in Europe and has the second-most obese population in the world (RCP, 2013). In England, 23% of all adults are clinically obese. It is acknowledged that often problems of overweight and obesity begin in childhood (DoH, 2011a), and currently almost a quarter of 4–5 year olds and a third of 10–11 year olds are overweight or obese (DoH, 2011c). Obesity is a major risk factor for Type 2 diabetes and heart disease, and people with severe mental illness are at increased risk of developing endocrine disorders (DoH, 2009).This, combined with the lifestyle and medication regimes of many clients with mental illness, should be of major concern to health care professionals, since all antipsychotic agents, both typical and atypical, increase the propensity to develop diabetes (Lambert *et al.*, 2003).

Diabetes increases the work demand of all the major organs, particularly the kidneys, and doubles the risk of developing heart disease (BHF, 2012). As obese people are five times more likely to develop Type 2 diabetes (DoH, 2011a) and as 40–62% of people with schizophrenia are obese or overweight, their risk of developing diabetes is substantially increased (Lambert *et al.*, 2003). Many factors contribute to a person's ability to stay at a healthy weight or succeed in losing weight. Lack of knowledge in relation to what constitutes a healthy diet, poor cooking skills, cost and availability of healthy food and limited opportunities or access to exercise may all contribute to obesity (DoH, 2006b). It must be acknowledged that action to address obesity may be much more difficult for those with mental illness and the clinical management of obesity cannot be viewed in isolation from the environment in which people live (DoH, 2006b). Recent evidence (RCP, 2013) suggests there is limited education regarding nutrition and obesity within the medical undergraduate curriculum and this is being addressed – similarly, nursing as a profession must therefore consider this a priority also.

Medical considerations for quality of care

National Institute for Health and Clinical Excellence (NICE) guidelines (DoH, 2009) provide best practice guidance for the care and treatment of schizophrenia and give equal weight to the need for physical health care, psychosocial and pharmacological interventions. The introduction of second generation, or atypical neuroleptics, has vastly improved the quality of life for those who experience positive symptoms associated with psychosis, compared to conventional antipsychotics such as Haloperidol and Chlorpromazine. Antipsychotics such as Risperidone, Quetiapine and, more recently, Clozapine address positive symptoms and have also proven to act upon the negative symptoms of psychotic illness, allowing service users to engage more effectively with others, increasing motivation and, as a consequence, promoting socialisation. However, though extrapyramidal side effects of atypical antipsychotics are less, other long-term side effects are evident, including rapid weight gain and its associated problems (DoH, 2009). Primary Care healthcare professionals are required to monitor the physical health of service users with schizophrenia annually, particularly in relation to the increased risk of cardiovascular disease associated with antipsychotic medication.

The prescribing of Clozapine as a treatment for schizophrenia is subject to strict guidelines. Nonresponse to sequential trials of at least two antipsychotics prior to the implementation of Clozapine regime is a requirement in the treatment of those with schizophrenia (DoH, 2009). This guideline highlights the major side effects of Clozapine, and stresses the benefit–risk ratio of its use. Both typical and atypical antipsychotics are associated with weight gain/obesity and its associated health implications, including diabetes. Atypical antipsychotics increase the risk of development of hyperlipidaema and diabetes (Lambert *et al.*, 2003), increasing the risk of chronic illness and premature mortality in those with severe forms of mental illness.

Emotional considerations for quality of care

Deliberate self-harm (DSH) can be defined as a nonfatal act in which an individual intentionally inflicts self-injury or self-poisoning (NICE, 2004; Hawton *et al.*, 2007). Common self-harm presentations include physical mutilation (e.g., cutting or burning), drug overdose/self-poisoning, jumping from a height and/or inserting objects into areas of soft tissue (e.g., limbs) or body cavities (Palmer, 2008). Statistics demonstrate that the UK has one of the highest rates of self-harm in Europe; though self-harm is not in itself a mental illness, there is a high correlation between self-harming and mental health (MHF), 2007. In the UK, cutting remains the second commonest self-harming behaviour after overdose (Gallup & Tulley, 2009). Though self-injury may have a close association with suicide, often the act of cutting, burning and using other methods of self-injury are often employed by individuals as a coping mechanism. They are attempts to relieve tension and communicate internal distress (MHF, 2007), and are used as a way of expressing emotional pain through physical means (Palmer, 2008). Within in-patient units, service users who had self-harmed did so privately, as a result of acute internal distress, conflict behaviours and following conflict with staff (James *et al.*, 2012). Those who self-injure are, for whatever reason, unable to communicate their needs effectively, and this group includes adolescents. It is estimated that 10–13% of 15–16 year olds have self-harmed (DoH, 2011b).

The decision to deliberately end life is always a tragic event, and it is recognised that there are certain high-risk groups within the UK population, that is, young and middle-aged men; people in the care of mental health services, including in-patients; and people with a history of self-harm (DoH, 2012a).

Social consideration for quality of care

Considerable stigma remains attached to a diagnosis of schizophrenia (DoH, 2009), and those in severe emotional and mental distress may experience feelings of hopelessness and feel suicide to be their only option. Though suicide is most common in the first few years following diagnosis (DoH, 2009), this may happen at any time, though feelings of hopelessness and despair are often precipitated and/or exacerbated by a person's social circumstances and adverse life events (DoH, 2012a). These include the breakdown of important relationships, unemployment and financial crisis (MHF, 2007). A recent increase in suicide rates may be associated with the current recession (DoH, 2012a), though it is generally accepted that suicide is often the consequence of a complex history of risk factors, and is precipitated as a result of a combination of factors. Since mental illness and physical illness are inextricably linked, and social factors may impact negatively on both, it is imperative that mental health nurses recognise and respond to the multiple factors which may contribute to the increased risk of suicide (DoH, 2012a). Many suicide attempts are closely associated with alcohol inebriation (Miller *et al.*, 2010) and any measures introduced to reduce alcohol dependence must surely be reflected in reduced suicide rates (DoH, 2012a).

Lifestyle considerations for quality of care

Though alcohol is legal and widely socially accepted, 4% of the UK population develop alcohol dependence, and experience the physical, psychological and social harmful effects of alcohol abuse (DoH, 2011d). Increased risk of alcohol dependence in adulthood is associated with consuming alcohol at an early age; additionally, early drinking is associated with mental and physical ill health, increased levels of violence, crime and accidental injury (Kiernan *et al.*, 2012). The toxicity and dependence-producing properties of alcohol result in an increased risk of developing cardiovascular and neuropsychiatric disorders, some cancers, and liver and pancreas disease.

Many people with mental illness use legal and illicit substances as part of a repertoire of coping mechanisms, finding that by indulging in such activities their problems temporarily diminish (Prymachuk, 2011). The toxins contained in tobacco affect the functionality of the heart, and increase blood pressure, doubling the risk of heart attack (BHF, 2012). Unhealthy habits often develop during the crucial developmental years. More than eight out of ten adults who smoke started smoking before the age of 19 (DoH, 2011a). Smoking is the single biggest preventable cause of early death and illness (DoH, 2011a). Adults with mental illness smoke 42% of all the tobacco used in England (Sainsbury Centre for Mental Health, 2011) and this places them at high risk of developing cardiovascular and respiratory disease. Additionally, smoking significantly increases the risk of stroke and the development of cancers of the mouth, throat, larynx, blood, lungs, stomach, pancreas, bladder and cervix (NIDA, 2010). Despite the perception of some health care professionals, smoking cessation treatments that work in the general population are equally effective in those with severe mental illness (Banham & Gilbody, 2010). Their study also suggests that mental state does not relapse if supported smoke cessation is initiated when the participants are mentally stable, indicating health promotion, signposting and referral to be central to the role of the mental health nurse, in line with the *Code of Conduct* (NMC, 2008).

The use of illicit substances is significantly higher in those with mental illness compared to the general population, and approximately 40% of people with psychosis misuse substances at some point in their lifetime, at least double the rate seen in the general population (DoH, 2011e). Reasons for this increased risk include genetic, neurological, developmental and environmental factors, as well as self-medication (Rassool, 2011). Environmental factors undoubtedly play a major role in the introduction of and sustained use of alcohol and illicit substances, demonstrated by the increased prevalence in areas of deprivation and social exclusion (Rassool, 2011). Physical complications as a result of illicit substance misuse are largely dependent on the type of substance being ingested, inhaled or injected, but include cardiovascular disease, particularly stroke, infected injection sites, respiratory disorders and liver cirrhosis.

Educational considerations for quality of care

In preparation for its future nursing workforce, the NMC has developed a competency framework within its Standards for *Pre-Registration Nursing* (NMC, 2010), which reinforces the need for a holistic approach to caring for clients with mental health problems. The framework requires that all nurses possess a broad knowledge of anatomy and physiology, in order to provide holistic, nonjudgemental caring and sensitive nursing care. The development of skills required to carry out comprehensive nursing assessment which consider physical, psychological and sociocultural factors is vital to the role of the Mental Health Nurse.

The Department of Health (DoH, 2011b) raised the expectation that mental health and physical health were of equal importance in the health agenda in the UK. In order to achieve wellbeing in our service users, we need to ensure the concept of holism is central to assessment and care delivery. Mental health professionals are legally and morally required to develop knowledge and skills in relation to caring for service users' physical health as well as addressing their mental health needs. The Mental Health Nurse must embrace the role of health promotion in order to meet the needs of service users who are unable, due to their mental state, to take action to promote and maintain their own physical health. The challenge lies in the need to develop the skills necessary to fulfil this vital aspect of the nursing role.

Practice-related considerations for quality of care

Acute service provisions, in particular, Emergency Departments (EDs) and Medical and Surgical inpatient wards, have been criticised for the level of 'relative neglect' that people with mental health issues encounter within these areas (AoMRC, 2008). As EDs come under increasing criticism, and increasing political pressure to meet various targets, including the 4-hour target (95% of patients need to be seen, treated, discharged or admitted within 4 hours), questions are being posed about the quality of the care being delivered (RCN, 2008). The aim of this section is to provide an overview of common mental health presentations to the emergency department, whilst exploring the role of ED staff in promoting health and wellbeing.

Emergency department and mental health

Emergency Departments (EDs/A&E/Casualty) are intrinsically unpredictable; people attend for a multitude of health issues ranging from minor injuries and ailments through to major trauma and life-threatening emergencies. However, it would be inaccurate to suggest that these departments deal solely with physical injury and illness; they are required to meet the 'full spectrum of human need' (Jones, 2008), regardless of the presenting problem ('whatever' and 'whoever'). As a result of this remit, nursing and medical staff working within the ED are required to have a breadth of knowledge which spans multiple specialities. The sometimes fast but always unpredict-able nature of the ED also demands efficient and thorough assessment skills to ensure care is prioritised, planned and managed appropriately (Wright *et al.*, 2012), and within a timely manner (4-hour targets). Adapting and applying these skills across the age continuum, from neonates through to older people, requires considerable skill and knowledge (Wright, 1993). However, questions have been posed in relation to the level and quality of care provided to those who attend with mental health issues (AoMRC, 2008; RCN, 2008; DoH, 2011b).

Self-harm is a subject which is often poorly understood by staff working within acute care areas, and can evoke mixed feelings and responses (Agulnik & Palmer, 2008). Self-harm accounts for around 150 000 presentations to the ED (NICE, 2004) each year within the UK, and represents a significant issue for EDs (Hadfield *et al.*, 2009), and Emergency Assessment Units (EAUs) alike (Holdsworth *et al.*, 2001). It is also one of the` most frequent reasons for acute medical admission to hospital (NICE, 2004). Hawton *et al*'s (2007) multicentre study of self-harm attendances to the ED concur with this observation and found that approximately 80% of all self-harm attendances could be attributed to self-poisoning, although Warncken & Dolan (2008) suggest this is more like 90%. However, it was noted that the most frequent method of self-poisoning could be attributed to Paracetamol overdose, although the method of self-poisoning altered with age (Paracetamol (younger age groups), antidepressants (middle-age groups), benzodiazepines/sedatives (older age groups) (Hawton *et al.*, 2007)).

Staff attitude towards people attending the ED with self-harm behaviour can have a major influence on health outcomes and the quality of treatment they receive (Mackay & Barrowclough, 2005). Despite the relatively high incidence of self-harm presentations, there still appears to be a lack of understanding and compassion in some departments. Some doctors described feelings of frustration when providing care to those attending with self-harm behaviour, especially those with repeated episodes of self-harm (Hadfield *et al.*, 2009). However, much of the reported frustration was around their inability to 'fix' the problem (i.e., stop future episodes of self-harm) (Marynowski-Traczyk & Broadbent, 2011). However, the ideology that health care is solely about treatment and cure, and the ability to 'fix' is not congruent with contemporary health models (Scriven, 2010; Evans *et al.*, 2011) nor is it aligned to the Recovery Model used within mental health (Marynowski-Traczyk & Broadbent, 2011). Hadfield *et al.* (2009) suggest ED doctors are constrained by the expectation that their focus should be on evidence-based treatments for physical treatments (treating the body). However, this reductionist approach fails to consider the mental and social aspects of health (Scriven, 2010; Evans *et al.*, 2011), and therefore is counterproductive for people attending with self-harm behaviour. Yet, aspects of the medical model are important within the ED; the vast majority of people attend EDs with physical injury or physical emergencies which require acute and often immediate intervention. It's understood, and recognised, that focusing upon physical needs alone would be reductionism; however, a balance is required to ensure the provision of care is focused upon the person as a whole; taking into account their individual needs within an environment of trust and respect, whilst meeting their immediate health needs (Marynowski-Traczyk & Broadbent, 2011).

Several misconceptions still exist around the reasons for self-harm behaviour; some health professionals believe it's a way of seeking attention or an attempt to manipulate (either situations or people), and feared that treating *them* would only serve to reinforce behaviour (Hadfield *et al.*, 2009). However, for the majority of people who engage in self-harm, it is a private event, something which may have been occurring for several years prior to seeking any form of help (Palmer, 2008), while for others, seeking help may be part of their coping mechanism. The intention is not to frustrate nor manipulate, but a way of communicating emotional pain through physical means (Palmer, 2008). Medical personnel within the ED were more pessimistic than their nursing counterparts around treating people with self-harm behaviour; much of this was linked to the belief that self-harm would be repeated (Mackay & Barrowclough, 2005).

Preventative considerations for quality of care

The importance of early diagnosis, intervention and treatment cannot be underestimated (DoH, 2011b). Equally, health professionals need to be aware of the risk factors associated with suicidal behaviour; these include individuals living alone or in isolation, having a drug or alcohol dependency, repeated episodes of self-harm and previous or current mental health problems (Cooper *et al.*, 2005; Murphy *et al.*, 2012). Professionals working with people with self-harming behaviour need to have the skills and knowledge to identify individuals who are vulnerable and high risk (one could argue this is all who attend with an episode of self-harm) to ensure they receive adequate care/intervention. A lack of compassion, poor assessment and negative attitudes could result in individuals not waiting for treatment, or failing to seek future help, which could result in tragic consequences (NICE, 2004). Negative and dismissive responses are unhelpful and may exacerbate existing emotions and add to the sense of guilt (Palmer, 2008). Dismissive or judgemental attitudes will only damage therapeutic relationships and may result in poorer outcomes when a person is at high risk of suicide (NICE, 2004).

Immediate Assessment within the ED is normally performed by the triage/assessment nurse (Warncken & Dolan, 2008). This initial encounter allows the nurse to ascertain the primary reason for attending, the history of the presenting illness/injury, past medical/psychiatric history and social/family history (Warncken & Dolan, 2008). Initial nursing priorities would depend upon the presenting problem; however, any issues with Airway, Breathing, or Circulation (A, B, C's) or any other immediate life-saving interventions would take immediate priority over psychological needs (NICE, 2004). However, it is also the role of the triage nurse to provide an immediate psychosocial assessment which considers immediate risk, capacity and willingness to wait for further assessment (NICE, 2004). Obtaining an accurate history of events is fundamental to the role of the triage nurse; information gained within this initial assessment will determine the length of wait; essentially it is a system of prioritising care based upon clinical need (Marsden, 2008). Any psychosocial assessment requires sensitivity, empathy, privacy and *time*. The latter is perceived to be in short supply within EDs. The need to ensure timely assessment, treatment and discharge or admission to a ward within the 4-hour national target is a real issue for many EDs.

The sheer volume of attendances to the ED necessitates rapid assessment skills and effective decision-making to maintain a constant flow through the department (Marsden, 2008); however, people with mental health issues present EDs with a different set of challenges to those with physical health issues (Wright *et al.*, 2012). History of events and presenting history can sometimes be ambiguous; this can require time and patience to ensure accuracy of events. However, this can be complicated further if the person is intoxicated with alcohol or drugs (Butler, 2012). As a result, mental health assessments can mean longer consultations; this can disrupt the natural flow and pace within the department, and effect the provision of care for others within the department (Marynowski-Traczyk & Broadbent, 2011). A number of further concerns have been raised in relation to the suitability of the ED environment for assessing and treating people who attend with mental health issues; most departments are unpredictable, noisy and at times volatile, which can cause anxiety and additional stress, resulting in poor client outcomes (Clarke *et al.*, 2007; Marynowski-Traczyk & Broadbent, 2011). The use of a quiet room, rather than the waiting area, is recommended (NICE, 2004) for those waiting for psychiatric assessment; however, this poses issues around safety, supervision and staff availability.

Recommendations from the Royal College of Psychiatrists and British Association for Accident and Emergency Medicine (2004) state that all 'A&E personnel should have adequate knowledge of mental health issues, and feel confident in making an initial assessment of people with mental health problems'; however, it is suggested (Holdsworth *et al.*, 2001; Hadfield *et al.*, 2009; Conlon & Tuathail, 2010) that this is not yet a reality. ED staff (nurses and doctors) have reported a deficiency in knowledge and skills (Conlon & Tuathail, 2010) and feel ill-prepared to manage the psychological aspects of care, suggesting emotional and psychological support was often difficult to provide, and an area in which they lacked experience (Hadfield *et al.*, 2009). The NICE clinical guidelines for self-harm (NICE, 2004) recognise the importance and need for adequate preparation and training for all staff working with people who self-harm; yet many still feel frustrated by the perceived lack of training and knowledge deficit (Hadfield *et al.*, 2009).

Conclusion

It is a stark reality that staff within the ED are restricted by time and targets; the 4-hour targets, a constant stream of physical and psychosocial admissions, and the worrying trend of GPs and hospital managers, allowing the ED to be utilised as a 'waiting room', have resulted in most departments 'fire-fighting' (crisis managing) most days. The expectation is that we can deliver high-quality care to all, regardless of presenting issues. EDs cannot say 'we have no beds', or 'we are full' and they cannot close admissions (unless under exceptional circumstances), and so the pressure mounts. This is not an attempt to justify or detract from the claims of poor care, or discriminatory practice; however, these are the complex realities which impact upon the standard and quality of care within the ED. There is a realisation that EDs have to improve the level of care which is provided to those who attend with mental health-associated illness/injuries, and this must be congruent with the level of care provided to those with physical health needs (AoMRC, 2008; DoH, 2011b). However, lack of education, lack of training, limited resources and environmental constraints all attribute to the current state of affairs.

References

Academy of Medical Royal Colleges (AoMRC) (2008) *Managing Urgent Mental Health Needs in Acute Trusts*. Academy of Medical Royal Colleges, London.

Agulnik, D. & Palmer, L. (2008) Reaching out. *Emergency Nurse*, **16** (5), 14–17.

Banham, L. & Gilbody, S. (2010) Smoking cessation in severe mental illness: what works? *Addiction*, **105**, 1176–1189.

Bee, P., Playle, J., Lovell, K., Barnes, P., Gray, R. & Keeley, P. (2008) Service user views and expectations of UK-registered mental health nurses: a systematic review of empirical research. *International Journal of Nursing Studies*, **45**, 442–457.

Brimblecombe, N., Tingle A., Tunmore, R. & Murrells, T. (2007) Implementing holistic practices in mental health nursing: a national consultation. *International Journal of Nursing Studies*, **44**, 339–348.

British Heart Foundation (BHF) (2012) *Quality and Outcomes Framework Guidance 2012–2013* [Online]. Available at http://www.bhf.org.uk. Accessed on May 4, 2013.

Brown, S., Inskip, H. & Barrowclough, B. (2000) Causes of excess mortality in schizophrenia. *British Journal of Psychiatry*, **177**, 212–217.

Butler, J. (2012) Self-harm. *Psychiatric Aspects of General Medicine*, **40** (12), 650–653.

Callaghan, A. (2004) Exercise: a neglected intervention in mental health care? *Journal of Psychiatric and Mental Health Nursing*, **11** (4), 476–483.

Clarke, D.E., Dusome, D. & Hughes, L. (2007) Emergency department from the mental health client's perspective. *International Journal of Mental Health Nursing*, **16**, 126–131.

Cohen, A. & Hove, M. (2001) *Physical Health of the Severe and Enduring Mentally Ill*. The Sainsbury Centre for Mental Health, London.

Conlon, M. & O'Tuathail, C. (2010) Measuring emergency department nurses' attitudes towards deliberate self-harm using the Self-Harm Antipathy Scale. *International Emergency Nursing*, **20**, 3–13.

Cooper, J., Kapur, N., Webb, R., *et al.* (2005) Suicide after deliberate self-harm: a 4-year cohort study. *American Journal of Psychiatry*, **162**, 297–303.

Crone, D. & Guy, H. (2008) 'I know it is only exercise, but to me it is something that keeps me going': a qualitative approach to understanding mental health service users' experiences of sports therapy. *International Journal of Mental Health Nursing*, **17**, 197–207.

Department of Health (DoH) (1990) *The NHS and Community Care Act*. The Stationery Office, London.

Department of Health (1999) *National Service Framework for Mental Health*. The Stationery Office, London.

Department of Health (2004) *National Service Framework for Coronary Heart Disease*. The Stationery Office, London.

Department of Health (2006a) *From Values to Action: The Chief Nursing Officer's Review of Mental Health Nursing*. The Stationery Office, London.

Department of Health (2006b) *NICE Obesity: The Prevention, Identification, Assessment and Management of Overweight and Obesity in Adults and Children*. The Stationery Office, London.

Department of Health (2009) *NICE Guidelines: Schizophrenia: Core Interventions in the Treatment and Management of Schizophrenia in Adults in Primary and Secondary Care*, The Stationery Office, London.

Department of Health (2011a) *Healthy Lives, Healthy People: Our Strategy for Public Health in England*. The Stationery Office, London.

Department of Health (2011b) *No Health without Mental Health*. The Stationery Office, London.

Department of Health (2011c) *Healthy Lives, Healthy People: A Call to Action on Obesity in England*, The Stationery Office, London.

Department of Health (2011d) *NICE Guidelines: Alcohol-use Disorders: Diagnosis, Assessment and Management of Harmful Drinking and Alcohol Dependence*. The Stationery Office, London.

Department of Health (2011e) *NICE Guidelines: Psychosis with Coexisting Substance Misuse: Assessment and Management in Adults and Young People*. The Stationery Office, London.

Department of Health (2012a) *Preventing Suicide in England: A Cross-Government Outcomes Strategy to Save Lives*. The Stationery Office, London.

Department of Health (2012b) *Compassion in Practice: Nursing Midwifery and Care Staff Our Vision and Strategy*. The Stationery Office, London.

Evans, D., Coutsaftiki, D. & Fathers, P.C. (2011) *Health Promotion and Public Health for Nursing Students*. Learning Matters, Exeter.

Gallup, R. & Tulley, T (2009) The person who self harms. In: *Psychiatric and Mental Health Nursing: The Craft of Caring* (ed. P.J. Barker), 2nd edn. pp. 191–199. Hodder Arnold, London.

Hadfield, J., Brown, D., Pembroke, L. & Hayward, M. (2009) Analysis of accident & emergency doctors' responses to treating people who self-harm. *Qualitative Health Research*, **19**, 755–765.

Hawton, K., Bergen, B., Caey, D., *et al.* (2007) Self-harm in England: a tale of three cities. *Social Psychiatry & Psychiatric Epidemiology*, **42**, 513–521.

Holdsworth, N., Belshaw, D. & Murray, S. (2001) Developing A&E nursing responses to people who deliberately self-harm: the provision and evaluation of a series of reflective workshops. *Journal of Psychiatric and Mental Health Nursing*, **8**, 449–458.

Howard, L. & Gamble, C. (2011) Supporting mental health nurses to address the physical health needs of people with serious mental illness in acute inpatient care settings. *Journal of Psychiatric and Mental Health Nursing*, **18**, 105–112.

James, K., Stewart, D., Wright, S. & Bowers, L. (2012) Self harm in adult inpatient psychiatric care: a national study of incident reports in the UK. *International Journal of Nursing Studies*, **49**, 1212–1219.

Johnstone, R., Nicol, K., Donaghy, M. & Lawrie, S. (2009) Barriers to uptake of physical activity in community-based patients with schizophrenia. *Journal of Mental Health*, **18** (6), 523–532.

Jones, G. (2008) Nursing in Emergency care. In: *Accident & Emergency theory into practice* (eds B. Dolan & L. Holt), Elsevier Limited, London.

Kiernan, C., Ni Fhearail, A. & Coyne, I. (2012) Nurses' role in managing alcohol misuse among adolescents. *British Journal of Nursing*, **21** (8), 474–478.

Lambert, T.J.R., Velakoulis, D. & Pantelis, C. (2003) Medical comorbidity in schizophrenia. *Medical Journal of America*, **178**, 67–70.

Mackay, N. & Barrowclough, C. (2005) Accident and emergency staff's perceptions of deliberate self-harm: attributions, emotions and willingness to help. *British Journal of Clinical Psychology*, **44**, 255–267.

Marsden, J. (2008) Nursing in emergency care. In: *Accident & Emergency theory into practice* (eds B. Dolan & L. Holt) Elsevier Limited, London.

Marynowski-Traczyk, D. & Broadbent, M. (2011) What are the experiences of emergency department nurses in caring for clients with a mental illness in the emergency department? *Australasian Emergency Nursing Journal*, **14**, 172–179.

Mental Health Foundation (MHF) (2007) *The Fundamental Facts: The Latest Facts and Figures on Mental Health*. Mental Health Foundation, London.

Miller, T.R., Teti, L.O., Lawrence, B.A. & Weiss, H.B. (2010) Suicide and life-threatening behaviour. *The American Association of Suicidology*, **40** (5), 492–499.

Murphy, E., Kapur, N., Webb, R., *et al.* (2012). Risk factors for repetition following self-harm in older adults: multicentre cohort study. *British Journal of Psychiatry*, **200**, 399–404.

Nash, M. (2011) Improving mental health service users' physical health through medication monitoring: a literature review. *Journal of Nursing Management*, **19**, 360–365.

National Institute for Health and Clinical Excellence (NICE) (2004) *Self-Harm: The Short-Term Physical and Psychological Management and Secondary Prevention of Self-Harm in Primary and Secondary Care*. The British Psychological Society, London.

National Institute for Drug Abuse (NIDA) (2010) *Drugs, Brains and Behaviour: The Science of Addiction* [Online]. Available at http://www.drugabuse.gov/publications/science-addiction/addiction-health Accessed on Oct 10, 2012.

Nursing & Midwifery Council (NMC) (2008) *Code of Conduct*. NMC, London.

Nursing & Midwifery Council (2010) *Standards for Pre-registration Nursing Education*. NMC, London.

Ohlsen, R. (2011) Schizophrenia: a major risk factor for cardiovascular disease. *British Journal of Cardiac Nursing*, **6** (5), 228–232.

Palmer, L. (2008) Helping people who self-harm. *Emergency Nurse*, **16** (3), 14–17.

Prymachuk, S. (2011) *Mental Health Nursing. An Evidence-Based Introduction*. Sage, London.

Rassool, G.H. (2011) *Understanding Addiction Behaviours: Theoretical & Clinical Practice in Health and Social Care*. Palgrave Macmillan, Basingstoke.

Royal College of Nursing (RCN) (2008) *A&E Nurses under Pressure to meet Four Hour Target* [Online]. Available at http://www.rcn.org.uk/newsevents/press_releases/uk/a_and_e_nurses_under_pressure_to_meet_four_hour_target. Accessed on Jan 28, 2013.

Royal College of Physicians (RCP) (2013) *Action on Obesity: Comprehensive Care for All. Report of A Working Party*. RCP, London.

Royal College of Psychiatrists & British Association for Accident and Emergency Medicine (2004) *Psychiatric Services to Accident and Emergency Departments*. Council Report CR118 RCP/BAAEM, London.

Sainsbury Centre for Mental Health (2011) *Physical Health of the Severe Enduring Mentally Ill a Training Pack for GP Educators*. Sainsbury Centre for Mental Health, London.

Scriven, A. (2010) *Promoting Health: A Practical Guide*, 6th edn. Elsevier, London.

Verhaeghe, N., De Maeseneer, J., Maes, L., Van Heeringen, C. & Annemans, L. (2011) Perceptions of mental health nurses and patients about health promotion in mental health care: a literature review. *Journal of Psychiatric and Mental Health Nursing*, **18**, 387–492.

Wand, T. & Murray, L. (2008) Let's get physical. *International Journal of Mental Health Nursing*, **17**, 363–369.

Warncken, B. & Dolan, B. (2008) Psychiatric emergencies. In: *Accident & Emergency Theory into Practice* (eds B. Dolan & L. Holt). Elsevier Limited, London.

Wright, B. (1993) Jack of all trades, master of none. *Accident & Emergency Nursing*, **1**, 1–2.

Wright, W., McGlen, I. & Dykes, S. (2012) Mental health emergencies: using a structured assessment framework. *Emergency Nurse*, **19** (10), 28–35.

Chapter 7

Strengths and Diversities: A Substance Misuse Perspective

Julie Wardell

Tees, Esk and Wear Valleys NHS Foundation Trust, UK

Introduction

Do you have much success? This is the most commonly asked question by everyone interested in this field, whether it be the lay person, family member, commissioner or government minister. However, this simple question belies the complex debates within this aspect of theory and practice. This chapter will explore the perspectives and approaches that are used within this field, by illustrating the models and interventions available for those who misuse substances. It will examine government strategy pertaining to policy and review in detail the current model for working within substance misuse, that is, the recovery model. It will then identify and explore the importance of working with individuals in a person-focused manner, enabling practitioners to elicit their goals, strengths and aspirations. It will highlight the need to work with individuals as part of families, broader social environments and communities. It will also review the perspectives, theories and models in this field, including strengths-based perspectives and motivational change models.

It is not uncommon for opiate users, that is, those who use heroin, to remain in treatment for ten years or more. This requires considerable commitment and resources from funders, users themselves and their families. Therefore, the primary focus of this chapter will be on opiate users and their treatment.

Care Planning in Mental Health: Promoting Recovery, Second Edition.
Edited by Angela Hall, Michael Wren and Stephan D. Kirby.
© 2013 John Wiley & Sons, Ltd. Published 2013 by John Wiley & Sons, Ltd.

Background to substance misuse

Substance misuse refers to the excessive consumption of and/or dependence on drugs, alcohol or volatile substances that leads a person to experience social, psychological, physical or legal problems which causes harm to themselves, their significant others and/or the wider community (NICE, 2007). Dependence is defined as a strong desire or sense of compulsion to take a substance, a difficulty in controlling its use, the presence of a physiological withdrawal state, tolerance of the use of the drug, neglect of alternative pleasures and interests and persistent use of the drug, despite harm to oneself and others (WHO, 2006). *The International Classification of Mental and Behavioural Disorders (ICD-10)* defines dependence as a 'cluster of psychological, behavioural and cognitive phenomena in which the use of substance takes on a much higher priority for a given individual than other behaviours' (WHO, 1992:70).

It has been reported that almost three million people in the UK use illicit drugs each year (Hoare & Moon, 2010) and it is estimated that in England 262 000 (less than 1% of the total population) people use the opioid, heroin (Hay *et al.*, 2010). The term 'opioid' refers to a substance derived from the poppy plant and includes morphine and codeine, as well as semisynthetic forms including heroin and synthetic compounds including methadone and buprenorphine (WHO, 2006.) Whilst opioid misuse occurs on a smaller scale than other drugs, it is associated with much greater rates of harm to individuals, their families and communities (NICE, 2008). Once an individual is dependent, opioid use is generally a chronic remitting condition, interspersed with periods of relapse and remission, often involving numerous treatment episodes over several years (Marsden *et al.*, 2004). For those who use opioids, most develop dependence in their late teens or early twenties and continue using over the next 10–30 years (NICE, 2008). Longitudinal data from the US showed that the average drug using career is 9.9 years (Joe *et al.*, 1990). Data from treatment providers show that the heroin-using population is ageing, with fewer young people becoming dependent on the drug. Those aged 40 years and above now make up the largest proportion of those newly presenting for treatment. It is likely that these individuals will be in poorer health, will engage in more dangerous injecting behaviour and are at greater risk of dying from overdose (NTA, 2010).

Heroin became a serious problem in Britain in the 1970s. Carnwath and Smith (2002) suggest that people only become dependent on heroin because it serves a useful function. They suggest that individuals may use heroin because they enjoy it, because it is an important feature of their social world, because it blots out painful memories or for a hundred different reasons. They carried out a research review which highlighted that heavy drugs and crime careers are embedded in the most disadvantaged communities. They suggest that this career is related to the increasing social exclusion of certain groups that has accompanied deindustrialisation, the decline of the welfare state and the rise of the consumer-based market economy. The clustering of drug use, crime, unemployment and deprivation in particular geographical areas has been irrefutably established in both American and British research. The current coalition government acknowledged that whilst dependence can affect anyone, there are those in society who are disproportionately likely to misuse substances, for example, those with a background of child-hood abuse, neglect, trauma or poverty (HM Government, 2010).

There is also a clear association between mental illness and drug and alco-hol dependence (HM Government, 2010). Those experiencing mental ill-health are at higher risk of substance misuse. Substantial evidence exists to connect poverty, ethnicity and gender causally to disabling distress. Psychological dis-tress is more prevalent in poorer communities than in more affluent ones. Impoverishment lowers self-esteem, reduces access to resources that sustain emotional wellbeing and exposes people to uncongenial living conditions, higher levels of crime and antisocial behaviour.

Approaches to substance misuse

It is important to acknowledge that individuals can and do cease their sub-stance misuse without any formal treatment (Biernacki, 1986). However, for many individuals, it is access to treatment that alters the course of their opioid dependence (NICE, 2008). Substance misuse interventions can be categorised into three broad approaches: 'harm reduction', 'maintenance-oriented treat-ments' and 'abstinence-oriented treatments'. All three approaches and their related treatments aim to prevent or reduce the harms resulting from the use of drugs and form part of treatment and recovery services.

Harm reduction interventions aim to prevent or reduce negative health or other consequences associated with drug misuse, whether to the person using drugs or, more widely, to society. With such approaches, it is not essen-tial for there to be a reduction in the drug use itself, although, of course, this may be one of the methods of reducing harm. Needle and syringe exchange services aim to reduce transmission of blood-borne viruses through the pro-motion of safer drug-injecting behaviour. Maintenance-oriented treatments in the UK context primarily refer to the pharmacological maintenance of peo-ple who are opioid dependent, through the prescription of opioid substitutes. This treatment aims to reduce or end their drug use and the consequential harms. Abstinence-oriented treatments aim to reduce an individual's level of drug use, with the ultimate goal of abstinence.

Care planning and keyworking are integral to successful treatment (NTA, 2006a) and recovery. Recovery care planning involves an agreed plan of action between the individual and service provider, identifying goals across four domains: substance misuse, health (physical and psychological), offending and social functioning (including housing, employment and relationships). The National Treatment Agency (NTA, 2006a) suggests that structured psychosocial interventions should be identified within the care plan. These are clearly defined, evidence-based interventions that assist the individual to make changes in their substance-misusing behaviour. These interventions are normally time limited and should be delivered by competent practitioners. Evidence-based psychosocial interventions include Cognitive Behaviour Therapy (CBT), Coping skills training, Relapse Prevention Therapy, Motivational interventions, Contingency management and Community reinforcement approaches (Wanigaratne *et al.*, 2005).

Government strategy and substance misuse

Prior to 1998, there was no coordinated approach to drug treatment and monitoring in the UK. In April 1998, the Labour government published a ten-year strategy for tackling drug misuse, *Tackling Drugs to Build a Better Britain* (HM Government, 1998). Their overarching aim was to develop and monitor an improved and robust drug treatment system. In order to do this, they set up the National Treatment Agency (NTA) for Substance Misuse, a special health authority within the NHS. Its purpose was to improve the availability, capacity and effectiveness of treatment for drug misusers in England. The objectives of the strategy were to enable people with drug problems to overcome them and live healthy and crime-free lives, thus protecting communities from drug-related antisocial and criminal behaviour. The plan to achieve this was to double the number of people in effective treatment from 1998 to 2008, by reducing waiting times and increasing the percentage of those successfully completing treatment or appropriately continuing treatment year on year (NTA, 2006a). The emphasis of the NTA was on delivering good quality drug treatments that improved the health of individuals, reduced drug-related offending, reduced the risk of death due to overdose and infections (including blood-borne infections) and improved social functioning.

In many ways the drug strategy of 1998 achieved what it set out to do. The drive to reduce waiting lists and to retain people in treatment resulted in much larger numbers entering treatment, significantly benefitting individuals and the communities in which they live (NTA, 2011). The drug treatment workforce grew significantly, enabling waiting times to be reduced from 9.1 weeks in December 2001 to 2.3 weeks by June 2005 (NTA, 2006a). Reviews have concluded that good quality drug treatment is effective at achieving the desired outcomes (HM Government, 2010).

In 2010, the coalition government produced a new drug strategy, *Reducing Demand, Restricting Supply, Building Recovery* (HM Government, 2010). The goal of the strategy was to reduce drug use and dependence and to enable individuals to leave treatment free of their drug of dependence. It suggested that there needed to be a shift from focusing primarily on reducing the harms caused by drug misuse to offering support for people to choose recovery as an achievable way out of dependency. Whilst they acknowledged that there are many thousands of people in receipt of substitute prescribing who have jobs, positive family lives and are no longer taking illegal drugs or committing crime, their critical observation was that 'for too many people currently on a substitute prescription, what should be the first step on the journey to recovery risks ending there' (HM Government, 2010:18). In pursuit of their goal to incentivise the system to deliver on recovery outcomes (payment by results), they allocated a significant proportion of funding based on individuals successfully exiting the treatment system. Individuals are therefore required to exit the treatment system free from all opioids, including all substitute prescribing (and not represent to services for at least 6 months), for this funding to be secured. These criteria will have significant implications for treatment services, and critics have argued that this will lead to a significant reduction in the funding for treatment systems, year on year.

Recovery and substance misuse

The recovery movement in the substance misuse field began in 1935 in the US with the mutual aid fellowship Alcoholics Anonymous (AA). However, the concept of recovery in mental health can be traced back as far as 1830 in Britain. The increasing ascendance of the community support concept and the practice of psychiatric rehabilitation of the 1980s laid the foundation for a 1990s vision of recovery for people with mental illness (Anthony, 1989).

There are many definitions of 'recovery' within both the mental health and substance misuse fields. Typically, definitions include the absence of prescribed medication (Watkins, 2007) and a socially inclusive lifestyle, including some employment activity and evidence of sustained independent living (Liberman *et al.*, 2002). However, these definitions have been criticised for not encompassing an individual's subjective experience of wellbeing and recovery (Davidson, 2003). Watkins (2007) suggested that recovery is about building a satisfying and meaningful life, as defined by the person themselves, and involves participation in the rights, roles and responsibilities of society, including being able to participate fully in family life and undertake work in a paid or a voluntary capacity.

The UK Drug Policy Commission Recovery Consensus Group (UKDPC, 2008), an independent, charitably funded body, reviewed the work on recovery and recognised that it can be achieved in many different ways. They suggest that recovery requires control over substances and to be free from the compulsion to use drugs. For some people, this will require abstinence from the problem substances or all substances. However, for others, it may mean abstinence supported by prescribed medication or consistently moderate use of some substances. They also believe that recovery must be voluntarily sustained in order for it to be long lasting, though they acknowledge that it may sometimes be initiated or assisted by 'coerced' or 'mandated' interventions within the criminal justice system. There can sometimes be a tendency by parents and observers to feel that forcible treatment may be the answer. This does not usually work, and threatening human freedom can increase individuals' resistance to change (Carnwath & Smith, 2002). The UKDPC (2008) believes that a broad 'vision' would be more useful than a 'definition', that is, "the process of recovery from problematic substance use is characterised by voluntarily sustained control over substance use which maximises health and wellbeing and participation in the rights, roles and responsibilities of society" (p. 6). They argue that the government's criteria for recovery based on successful exits from treatment suggests that substitute prescribing is incompatible with recovery. Indeed, McDermott (2010) highlights that nobody would expect individuals with schizophrenia or diabetes to stop taking their medication whilst they were still deriving benefits from it. In an interim report published by the NTA (2011), Professor John Strang concluded that the medication component can be significant in recovery and that the compatibility lies in ensuring that all individuals in receipt of a substitute prescription engage in recovery activities. He highlighted the diversity and complexity of both substance misuse and the needs of substance misusers and he suggested the need for all individuals to have regular reviews of progress, to enable the practitioner and individual to assess continuing and changing needs and appropriate responses. He suggested the use of the Treatment Outcome Profile (TOP) which has been specifically developed and validated for this purpose (Marsden *et al.*, 2008).

Personalising recovery in substance misuse

The diversity of experience regarding the recovery debate in substance misuse poses a challenge to anyone seeking to define it. Many authors suggest that the term 'recovery' is not a particularly helpful term for what is essentially a process of growth and change. Watkins (2007) suggests that such a process is not a destination but an ongoing journey. The trans-theoretical model (cycle of change) proposed by Prochaska and DiClemente (1982) predicts that substance misusers pass through five stages of change on their way to resolving the problem: 'Precontemplation', 'Contemplation', 'Determination', 'Action' and 'Maintenance'. The model is primarily concerned with motivation to change and the processes that lead to change. It also highlights the crucial task of matching interventions to the individual's readiness to change. Motivation has been viewed as fundamental to successful change attempts and, because of this, motivational interviewing has been hailed an important advance in the treatment of substance misuse (Heather, 1992). Motivational Interviewing is built on a fundamental objection to the traditional disease-oriented model of motivation that describes motivation as a characteristic of the individual (Barber, 1995). Devised by Miller (1983), it argues that the motivational state can be influenced (Miller & Rollnick, 1991) and that strategies should be more persuasive than coercive and more supportive than argumentative.

Many authors argue that treatment effectiveness may be as much about how treatment is delivered as it is about what is delivered (NTA, 2006b). As has been shown in the field of mental health, the development of recovery-oriented services requires a different relationship between people who use services and professionals and thus there will be many challenges in adopting this approach (Shepherd *et al.*, 2008). Booth *et al.* (1998) suggest that whilst choice may be a good thing in itself, it can also improve the prospects for a successful outcome. Miller (1989) argues that 'self-matching' is more likely to lead to completion of treatment. Individuals are more likely to carry through a course of action they have chosen for themselves, rather than one that has been chosen for them (Deci & Ryan, 1985). The recovery care plan must be developed collaboratively so that it is personally 'owned' and meaningful to the individual (NTA, 2011). Individuals should be provided with the relevant information to be able to make informed choices, including taking risks. The right of people to make choices about risk should be respected and promoted with the aim of achieving positive ends (Titterton & Smart, 2012). Watkins (2007) argues that as individuals know the most about themselves, relationships need to be more collaborative and facilitative rather than authoritative. In a recovery-oriented environment, there should not be an expert and a user; instead, the roles should be interchangeable. This may mean that practitioners need to learn new skills and to adapt roles to strengthen the leadership positions of individuals and their families (Best *et al.*, 2009).

There is an accumulation of evidence from psychotherapy research showing that some therapists achieve better results than others. It suggests an outcome variance of between 9 and 50% is accounted for by therapist characteristics (Crits-Christoph & Mintz, 1991). Messer and Wampold (2002) even suggest that therapist characteristics can be more powerful than the specific treatment. Diclemente *et al.* (2003) suggest that the therapeutic relationship may be critical to the change process. Prochaska and DiClemente (1984) described 'helping relationships' which entice individuals to make changes by conveying that he/she is valued and respected. Rogers (1951) claimed that truly healing relationships bloomed from the qualities of caring, empathy, positive regard, genuineness and respect. Similarly, Najavits and Weiss (1994) characterise more effective therapists as empathic, supportive, goal-directed, understanding, encouraging autonomy and effective at using external resources. They identified that less effective therapists are characterised as psychologically distant, overwhelming, belittling, controlling and self-interested.

Strengths-based practice in substance misuse

In recent years, strengths-based approaches have been increasingly used within substance misuse services. Strengths-based practitioners advise the avoidance of coercion, threats or the use of mythologising or stereotypical language such as attention seeker or nuisance. Saleebey (2006) suggests the need to move away from the problem or pathology perspective. He argues that accentuating problems creates a wave of pessimistic expectation of, and predictions about, the individual and his/her environment, and the capacity to cope with that environment. Furthermore, he argues that these labels can alter how individuals see themselves and how others see them and can seep into an individual's identity. However, he acknowledges that 'starting where the client is' requires an initial acknowledgement of the nature of the problem, as identified by the individual. Strengths-focused practitioners believe that the retelling of a problem-based narrative can serve to reinforce a 'stuck story' where the person hits the same wall each time. The 'unsticking' of the story comes through careful and attentive listening to clues provided by individuals about their family and friends, social connections, personal resources, their capacities and dreams for a better life. The eventual linking of their aspirations with existing and new resources provides the energy to build a life beyond the problem. Creating the imaginative world where aspirations can be converted to practical goals is a powerful strategy for establishing plans to reach those dreams. Change can only come about through understanding of, and collaboration with, the individual's aspirations, goals, perceptions and strengths. Strengths include what people have learned about themselves, their personal qualities, traits and virtues as well as in their spiritual, cultural and personal stories. Studies have shown that a switch from pathology to strengths meant that many people who had been categorised as 'hopeless cases' began to make improvements in their lives, for example, gaining employment and making new friends (Rapp & Weinstein, 1989; Kisthardt, 1993; Rapp & Chamberlain, 1995).

In many ways, the strengths perspective shares its underpinnings with solution-focused therapy. However, rather than a focus on goal setting, Solution-Focused Therapy emphasises solution finding through a strategy of purposeful questions that are intended to develop a detailed picture of a future beyond the problem. Also, the degree to which problems are acknowledged is a key difference between the two philosophies. Solution-focused therapy advocates skipping the broader 'assessment' that invariably includes details about and history of problems. In essence, it regards individuals in the light of what they have done well, those times that the problem has not been apparent or those times when exceptions to difficulty have occurred. Furthermore, the individual's goals and visions are the centrepiece of the work to be done. Solution-focused therapists concentrate on how things would be positively different. Perhaps the most well-known question that connects individuals with solutions is the Miracle question, a very effective way to invite conversations about goals (DeJong & Berg, 2001). Individuals are asked to imagine that their problem has been miraculously solved whilst they were sleeping. They are helped to create a picture of a 'reality' that they are capable of achieving and motivated to take action to create. Since it is their plan, they are more likely to view the plan as viable; to take action on the plan; and to gain a sense of competence, dignity, and worth through experiencing their own success (DeJong & Miller, 1995).

A second type of question used by the solution-focused model is the 'exception' question. The question flows out of the assumption that all problems in social systems have exceptions, and those exceptions involve strengths, resources and abilities (Berg, & Miller, 1992). For example, 'when were you tempted to take drugs yet didn't do so?' The effect is to highlight that the individual has the ability to do something different as well as to reconnect with the intention to make positive choices. Asking questions that assume that people have resources which help them achieve their goals not only highlights strengths and abilities but also directly links together their intentions, goals, and abilities for purposeful action.

The literature on resilience also provides conceptual and clinical ground for employing an individual's strengths as a central part in the helping process. Resilience is a process of continuing growth and articulation of capacities, knowledge, insight and virtues derived through meeting the demands and challenges of one's world. It is the ability to bear up in spite of ordeals. Benard (1994) states that 'using resilience as the knowledge base for practice creates a sense of optimism and hope'. Practitioners should never underestimate the sway of hope and the belief in the potential of people to grow. The placebo effect highlights the power of hope, positive expectation and belief in the healing ministration. As Saleebey (2006) points out, in many clinical trials, up to 60% of patients in placebo groups experienced therapeutic outcomes.

Involvement and engagement in recovery from substance misuse

Many individuals who have misused substances have identified remarkable strength and resilience to survive or to maintain their lifestyle under incredibly difficult circumstances. However, the ability to harness this to enable them to achieve their hopes and dreams has often been a complex process. These individuals are diverse and often have physical and mental health problems as well as social problems, requiring complex interventions (NTA, 2011). Due to their preoccupation with drug taking and the behaviours associated with this, they may have become estranged from family and friends, be poorly housed or not involved in activities that they find meaningful. To enable them to make these changes to their lives, they are likely to require support from their families as well as broader social systems.

The government strategy (DoH, 2011) uses the term 'recovery capital' to describe what is required to sustain recovery. One way to build capital is to establish opportunities to strengthen or develop individuals' social networks, involving family and friends. This may require facilitated meetings or even mediation services. Evidence shows that treatment is more likely to be effective, and recovery to be sustained, where families, partners and carers are closely involved (Copello *et al.*, 2005). Mutual Aid is a long-established successful means of support for individuals in recovery. Narcotics Anonymous and the more recently established Smart Recovery are peer-led meetings enabling individuals to benefit from support from others who have similar shared experiences.

Encouraging and enabling individuals to develop appropriate alternatives to substance misuse can be a complex process. It involves individuals replacing the enjoyment they sought from drug taking, as well as developing their confidence, self-esteem and capabilities to enable them to achieve a level of coping that means that they no longer need or want to blot out painful memories. For some people, this will involve obtaining employment, but for many others, years of substance misuse can present a significant barrier (Hay & Bauld, 2008). For many, it will require a staged approach, which may include support, training, volunteering or peer mentoring. Peer Mentoring has dual benefits for both mentors and mentees and can provide the opportunity to improve interpersonal skills. It can also help to build confidence, self-esteem and encourage a positive participation in society.

Recovery is also about empowerment (Ahern & Fisher, 2001) and providing the right conditions that people need to regain power over their lives and to make progress (Best *et al.*, 2009). For some individuals, the opportunity to become involved in the delivery of treatment or aftercare services is an ideal way to achieve this. It enables them to develop skills, confidence and self-esteem in areas where they have experience. It benefits service development by incorporating their views, which can help to develop and improve services. They can also act as a valuable resource to involve other individuals who have proven difficult to engage. Furthermore, involving individuals in recovery services offers a visible example that recovery is possible. This can act as a positive example to their peers to encourage them into recovery activities. McDermott (2010) highlights the emergence of individuals 'in recovery' in the user-involvement scene as one of the biggest changes in substance misuse in the last decade. It is important to acknowledge that there has also been an increasing willingness of employers to recruit these individuals as volunteers, recovery mentors or paid workers.

The development of these advancements on a significantly wider scale will require fundamental changes to how individuals as well as systems work in unison to achieve this. This would include family and friends, peers, mutual aid, treatment systems, criminal justice agencies, housing agencies and training and employment agencies. There would be a necessity for the statutory sector, voluntary sector, social enterprises and commissioners to work more closely together. It would require innovative working in partnership and commitment to overcoming barriers that lead to duplication and individuals missing out on seamless, joined-up services. Services would need to sign up to information-sharing protocols, which would enable them to implement single documents for assessment and recovery care planning. There should be regular meetings where recovery plans are developed and reviewed. Also, individuals and their families should be involved at all levels, including in commissioning and policymaking.

Evaluating recovery from substance misuse

So do we have much success? How do we measure success with this complex and diverse group of individuals who require complex interventions? Drug treatment has been proven to be successful on many fronts in the past 20 years. National and international evidence consistently shows that good treatment is highly effective in reducing illegal drug misuse, improving the health of drug misusers, reducing drug related offending, reducing the risk of death due to overdose, reducing the risk of death due to infections (including blood-borne virus infections) and improving social functioning. However, drug use involves risks and unfortunately there were 1784 substance misuse deaths in England and Wales in 2010 of which approximately 50% can be attributed to opioid use (Office for National Statistics, 2010).

So do people recover? Significant numbers of individuals successfully complete treatment from heroin use every year. The numbers of individuals using heroin reduced by 11 000 in 2008/2009 (Hoare & Moon, 2010). For most people recovery is a gradual process which may take years, during which time individuals pass through the 'cycle of change' several times. Relapse is common, sometimes in the form of short-term lapses and other times for longer periods. Fortunately, progress is cumulative between relapses and the length of the last period of abstinence is the best predictor of the next (Carnwath & Smith, 2002). The challenge is to ensure that high aspirations are maintained in the face of relapse and it is important that practitioners regularly consider whether to change the balance between promoting reducing harms and promoting the overcoming of dependence (NTA, 2011). This requires assessing the balance between risk management and enabling clients to improve their lives.

People can only recover if they have the belief and desire to do so and NTA (2010) suggests that individuals who have successfully completed treatment should be visible to current users in treatment. Recruiting these individuals as volunteers, recovery mentors or paid workers is an important way to do this.

Conclusion

Drug treatment saves lives, improves health and wellbeing and leads to recovery for a significant number of people. Services are committed to offering prompt access to high quality, appropriate interventions for people who misuse substances across all three approaches: 'harm reduction', 'maintenance-oriented' and 'abstinence-oriented treatments'. The increasing consensus and momentum towards recovery-orientated treatment services, which place the individual at its core, signals a real opportunity for a radical shift to improving outcomes for those affected by the problems of substance misuse. There is also a real shift towards involving and engaging individuals in substance misuse services, with the use of peer mentors and volunteers as well as progress in developing information-sharing protocols and shared processes.

Opioid treatment will continue to be challenging due to the complex needs of individuals as well as the chronically remitting condition of dependence. A further challenge lies in the timescales expected for changes to occur. There is an acknowledgement that delivering recovery-oriented treatment is complex and that it may take time for systems to fully reorientate to achieve the best balance between reduction of negatives and the accrual of positives for individuals. There is also considerable uncertainty and concern regarding the impact of payment by results on services, especially the outcomes-based funding criteria for successful treatment exits. Further work, involving individuals and their families, is needed to consider how we can best measure recovery and how this might be used to improve service provision for the future.

There is increasing agreement regarding what constitutes recovery, which includes being free from drugs of dependence, maximising health and wellbeing and building a satisfying life. There is also a shared understanding of the essential components required to sustain recovery such as strengthening social networks, mutual aid, peer support and paid or voluntary employment. However, an increase in the number unemployed means that there is a reduction of opportunities for a group already stigmatised.

There is still work to be done in developing a 'recovery-oriented work-force' and on changing relationships which enable the empowerment of individuals to regain power over their lives. There should be more emphasis on developing motivation, strengths and solutions rather than focusing on problems.

Recovery places the individual at its core, but the onus is on broader social systems and practitioners to ensure that a recovery-conducive environment is fostered. Nevertheless, there is a real opportunity for radical improvement in outcomes for those affected by the problems of substance misuse. Recovery requires a change of ethos from substance misuse services, in that it requires practitioners to consider and improve their practice in strengths-based and solution-focused approaches, with a focus on the future. Recovery requires the building of aspirations and hope from the individual their families and those providing services and support (UKDPC, 2008). But it is the hopes, expectations and dreams, the promise of possibilities of a better life, a different path, and the mobilising of their resources and assets that spur many to action. These are often unused or forgotten by the user or ignored by the professional, due to preoccupation with the label, at the expense of not 'seeing the whole person' which is detrimental to the recovery journey.

References

Ahern, L. & Fisher, D. (2001) Recovery at your own pace. *Journal of Psychosocial Nursing and Mental Health Services*, **39**, 4.

Anthony, W.A. (1989) Recovery from mental illness: the guiding vision of the mental health service in the 1990s. *Psychosocial Rehabilitation Journal*, **16** (4), 11–23.

Barber, J.G. (1995) *Social Work with Addictions*. Macmillan, London.

Benard, B. (1994) Applications of resilience. Paper presented to *A National Institute on Drug Abuse Conference on the Role of Resilience in Drug Abuse, Alcohol Abuse and Mental Illness*, Washington, DC.

Berg, I.K. & Miller, S. (1992) *Working with the Problem Drinker: A Solution Focused Approach*. Norton, New York.

Best, D., Groshkova, T. & McTague, P. (2009) The politics of recovery. *Druglink*, **24** (4), 14–19.

Biernacki, P. (1986) *Pathways from Heroin Addiction. Recovery without Treatment*. Temple University Press, Philadelphia.

Booth, P.G., Jones, A., Taylor, N. & Murphy, D. (1998) Treatment setting and treatment outcome in alcohol dependency: residential and day-care options compared. *Health and Social Care in the Community*, **6**, 251–259.

Carnwath, T. & Smith, I. (2002) *Heroin Century*. Routledge, London.

Copello, A., Velleman, R. & Templeton, L. (2005) Family interventions in the treatment of alcohol and drug problems. *Drug and Alcohol Review*, **24**, 369–385.

Crits-Christoph, P. & Mintz, J. (1991) Implications of therapist effects for the design and analysis of comparative studies of psychotherapies. *Journal of Consulting and Clinical Psychology*, **59**, 20–26.

Davidson, L. (2003) *Living Outside Mental Illness: Qualitative Studies of Recovery in Schizophrenia*. University Press, New York.

Deci, E.L. & Ryan, R.M. (1985) *Intrinsic Motivation and Self-Determination in Human Behaviour*. Plenum Press, New York.

DeJong, P. & Berg, I.K. (2001) *Interviewing for Solutions*, 2nd edn. Wadsworth, Belmont.

DeJong, P. & Miller, S.D. (1995) How to interview for client's strengths. *Social Work*, **40**, 729–736.

Department of Health (DoH) (2011) *No Health without Mental Health: A Cross Government Mental Health Outcomes Strategy for People of All Ages*. Office of Public Sector Information, London.

Diclemente, C.C., Carroll, K.M., Miller. W.R., Connors, C.J. & Donovan, D.M. (2003) A look inside treatment: therapist effects, the therapeutic alliance, and the process of intentional behaviour change. In: *Treatment Matching in Alcoholism* (eds T.F. Babor & F.K. Del Boca), pp. 166–183. Cambridge University Press, Cambridge.

Hay, G. & Bauld, L. (2008) *Population Estimates of Problematic Drug Users in England Who Access DWP Benefits: A Feasibility Study*, DWP Working Paper No. 46. Department for Work and Pensions, London.

Hay, G., Gannon, M., Casey J. & Millar, T. (2010) *Estimates of the Prevalence of Opiate Use and/or Crack Cocaine Use, 2008/09: Sweep 5 Report*. National Treatment Agency, London.

Heather, N. (1992) Addictive disorders are essentially motivational problems. *British Journal of Addiction*, **8**, 825–835.

HM Government (1998) *Tackling Drugs to Build a Better Britain: The Government's 10-Year Strategy for Tackling Drug Misuse April 98 Cm 3845*. HM Government, London.

HM Government (2010) *Drug Strategy: Reducing Demand, Restricting Supply, Building Recovery: Supporting People to Live a Drug Free Life*. HM Government, London.

Hoare, J. & Moon, D. (2010) *Drug Misuse Declared: Findings from the 2009/10 British Crime Survey England and Wales Home Office Statistical Bulletin 13/10*. Home Office, London.

Joe, G.W. Chastain, R.L. & Simpson, D.D. (1990) Length of careers. In: *Opioid Addiction and Treatment: A 12-Year Follow-Up* (eds D.D. Simpson & S.B Sells), pp. 103–120. Robert E. Krieger Publishing Company, Malabar.

Kisthardt, W. (1993) The impact of the strength's model of case management from the consumer perspective. In: *Case Management: Theory and Practice* (eds M. Harris & H.C. Bergman), pp. 112–125. Longman, New York.

Liberman, R.P., Kopelowicz, A., Ventura, J. & Gutkind D (2002) Operational criteria and factors related to recovery from schizophrenia. *International Review of Psychiatry*, **14**, 256–272.

Marsden, J., Farrell, M., Bradbury, C., *et al.* (2008) Development of the treatment outcomes profile. *Addiction*, **103** (9), 1450–1460.

Marsden, J. Strang, J. Lavoie, D., Abdulrahim, D., Hickman, M. & Scott, S. (2004) Drug misuse. In: *Health Care Needs Assessment: The Epidemiologically Based Needs Assessment Reviews* (eds A. Stevens, J. Raftery, J. Mant & S. Simpson), pp. 367–450. Radcliffe Medical Press, Abingdon.

McDermott, P. (2010) Use your head. *Druglink*, **25** (4), 26–27.

Messer, S.B. & Wampold, B. (2002) Let's face facts: common factors are more potent than specific therapy ingredients. *Clinical Psychology: Science and Practice*, **9**, 21–25.

Miller, W.R. (1983) Motivational interviewing with problem drinkers. *Behavioural Psychotherapy*, **1**, 147–172.

Miller, W.R. (1989) Matching individuals with interventions. In: *Handbook on Alcoholism Treatment Approaches: Effective Alternatives* (eds R.K. Hester & W.R. Miller), Pergamon Press, New York.

Miller, W.R. & Rollnick, S. (1991) *Motivational Interviewing. Preparing People to Change Addictive Behaviour*. The Guildford Press, London.

Najavits, L.M. & Weiss, R.D. (1994) Variations in therapist effectiveness in the treatment of patients with substance misuse disorders: an empirical review. *Addiction*, **89**, 679–688.

National Institute for Health and Clinical Excellence (NICE) (2007) *Interventions to Reduce Substance Misuse among Vulnerable Young People (PH4)*. NICE, London.

National Institute for Health and Clinical Excellence (2008) *National Clinical Practice Guideline Number 51: Drug Misuse: Psychological Interventions*. The British Psychological Society and The Royal College of Psychiatrists, London.

National Treatment Agency (NTA) (2006a) *Models of Care for Treatment of Adult Drug Misusers: Update 2006*. DoH, London.

National Treatment Agency (2006b) *Review of the Effectiveness for Alcohol Problems*. DoH, London.

National Treatment Agency (2010) *Drug Treatment in 2009/10*. NTA, London.

National Treatment Agency (2011) *Recovery-Orientated Drug Treatment. An Interim Report by Professor John Strang, Chair of the Expert Group*. NTA, London.

Office for National Statistics (2010) *Deaths Related to Drug Poisoning in England and Wales, 2010*. The Stationery Office, London.

Prochaska, J.O. & DiClemente, C.C. (1982) Transtheoretical therapy: toward a more integrative model of change. *Psychotherapy: Theory, Research and Practice*, **19**, 276–278.

Prochaska, J.O. & DiClemente, C.C. (1984) *The Transtheoretical Approach: Crossing the Traditional Boundaries of Therapy*. Dow Jones-Irwin, Homewood.

Rapp, C.A. & Chamberlain, P. (1995) Case management services to the chronically mentally Ill. *Social Work*, **30** (5), 417–422.

Rapp, C.A. & Wintersteen, R. (1989) The strengths based model of case management: Results from twelve demonstrations. *Psychosocial Rehabilitation Journal*, **13**, 23–32.

Rogers, C. (1951) *Client Centred Therapy: Its Current Practice, Theory and Implementations*. Houghton Mifflin, Chicago.

Saleebey, D. (ed.) (2006) *The Strengths Perspective in Social Work Practice*. Pearson Education, London.

Shepherd, G., Boardman, J. & Slade, M. (2008) *Making Recovery a Reality*. Sainsbury Centre for Mental Health, London.

Titterton, M. & Smart, H. (2012) Getting to grips with risk. *Professional Social Work*.

UK Drug Policy Commission Recovery Consensus Group (UKDPC) (2008) *A Vision of Recovery*. UKDPC, London.

Wanigaratne, S., Davis, P., Pryce, K. & Brotchie J. (2005) *The Effectiveness of Psychological Therapies on Drug Misusing Clients*. NTA, London.

Watkins, P.N. (2007) *Recovery: A Guide for Mental Health Practitioners*. Churchill Livingstone, London.

World Health Organization (WHO) (1992) *The ICD-10 Classification of Mental and Behavioural Disorders*. World Health Organization, Geneva.

World Health Organization (2006) *Lexicon of Alcohol and Drug Terms Published by the World Health Organization* [Online]. Available at http://www.who.int/substance_abuse/terminology/who_lexicon/en/. Accessed on May 27, 2013.

Section 2

Managing

Chapter 8

The Legal and Ethical Landscape

Charlotte Chisnell and Gordon J. Mitchell
Teesside University, UK

Contemporary practice in mental health is underpinned by both compulsory powers to detain, and a responsibility to advocate on behalf of, people who are vulnerable and socially excluded. It could be argued that mental health policy owes much to the legacy of its history, and the relationship between past and current practice should not be underestimated. Gould and Martin (2012) suggest that the historical context of mental health legislation represents a pendulum between medical paternalism and legalism, and within this conflict social work assumes the role of arbitrator. The provision of mental health services has moved from the view that treatment should mean institutionalisation and containment to the rhetoric of community care. More recently, the focus has shifted to needs-based assessments, campaigns from users of services and their relatives for better services, social inclusion and parity of esteem.

The intention of the chapter is to provide an overview of the recent changes that have been made in relation to mental health legislation by the 2007 Mental Health Act (MHA) (DoH, 2007) and the Mental Capacity Act (MCA) 2005 (DoH, 2005), and to discuss whether these changes are compatible with recent Government policy drivers such as, *No Health Without Mental Health*, (DoH, 2011), which endorses a recovery model of service provision and enablement. This strategy sets out six key objectives to improve outcomes for people with mental health issues:

- More people will have good mental health;
- More people with mental health problems will recover;
- More people with mental health problems will have good physical health;
- More people will have a positive experience of care and support;

Care Planning in Mental Health: Promoting Recovery, Second Edition.
Edited by Angela Hall, Michael Wren and Stephan D. Kirby.
© 2013 John Wiley & Sons, Ltd. Published 2013 by John Wiley & Sons, Ltd.

- Fewer people will suffer avoidable harm;
- Fewer people will experience stigma and discrimination.

(DoH, 2011)

Review of the Mental Health Act 1983

Following growing criticism of care within the community and mental health provision, New Labour began to develop its 'Third Way' policies in mental health services, whereupon partnership and collaboration were seen as key features of this approach. The internal market was to be replaced with 'integrated care', but the separation between planning/commissioning and provision was to remain. Alongside these social policy changes New Labour instigated a review of existing mental health legislation, the MHA 1983. The White Paper, Reforming the MHA, (DoH, 2000a) met with considerable opposition from a diverse alliance of interested parties, including the Royal College of Psychiatry, and service user and carer organisations. The main political drivers for reform of the mental health legislation focused on both safeguarding patient rights within a framework of managing risk (DoH, 2000a).

There was a cautious welcome from key stakeholders to the outline proposals, the Sainsbury Centre for Mental Health, although not as critical as many, about the new proposals argued that, 'at the heart of this issue is an apparent confusion about the required outcomes from mental health policy – whether this is aimed at enabling patients to recover from their mental illness or whether it is aimed at securing public safety' (Sainsbury Centre for Mental Health, 2007).

The proposed legislative reforms were undertaken within a backdrop of growing recognition that people with mental health issues are often the most marginalised and stigmatised groups in society. More attention began to be paid to the service user voice and the importance of overcoming barriers to social inclusion. Within this context, the principles of recovery began to be recognised and supported by several mental health professionals and within policy documents such as, *Our Health, Our Care, Our Say* (DoH, 2006), promoting a new rationale for mental health services.

In May 2006, the government announced it was going to proceed by introducing amendments to the existing MHA 1983 rather than introduce a new bill. The MHA 2007 was given Royal Assent in October 2007, and was fully introduced in October 2008. However, despite support for service user involvement and recognition of recovery-orientated services, these principles are often juxtaposed with the medical model, which has historically dominated the provision of mental health services and legislation (Table 8.1).

Table 8.1 A summary of the main changes.

Changes	Amendment to 1983 Act
Single definition of mental disorder	Proposals made for amending the definition of mental disorder to remove the separate categories under the MHA (1983) definition becomes 'any disorder or disability of mind' (section 1)
Appropriate treatment test	Current criteria for detention is to remain, with a stipulation that medical treatment must be available, but the 'treatability' test is to be abolished.
	Treatment appropriate to the person's mental disorder and circumstances must be actually available (section 3)
New definition of medical treatment	The old definition in section 145 was: 'medical treatment includes nursing, and also includes care, habilitation and rehabilitation under medical supervision'.
	Under the MHA 2007 changes, section 145 states that: 'medical treatment includes nursing, psychological intervention and specialist mental health habilitation, rehabilitation and care'
Two new professional roles	ASWs to be replaced by AMHP, approved by, but not necessarily employed by, the Local Authority. Responsible Medical Officer to be replaced by the Clinical Supervisor and could include Psychologists, Nurses, Social Workers, but must be trained and 'approved clinicians' (section 114A and section 142A)
Right to displace nearest relative	Broader grounds to be introduced for patient to displace the Nearest Relative (NR), for example, where NR is abusive to patient. Civil Partners to be recognised as NR. People who are receiving compulsory treatment can go to court to displace their nearest relative (section 29)
New ECT safeguards	A person with capacity who does not want ECT cannot be forced to have it (section 58A)
Supervised community Treatment	Replaces supervised discharge (section 17A–section 17G)
	A move from the proposed nonresidential orders to 'Supervised Community Treatment Orders' (SCTO). Significantly, these were restricted to patients compulsorily detained under section 3 of the MHA. The Clinical Supervisor must consult with an AMHP when making the order. The SCT order could include requirements, for example, recontact and there were set criteria for recalling the patient to hospital for treatment, which had to be agreed by the Clinical Supervisor and AMHP.

(Continued)

Table 8.1   *(Continued)*

Changes	Amendment to 1983 Act
Mental Health Tribunals	Earlier access to Mental Health Review Tribunals for appeals and review Duty of Hospital Managers to refer cases to the Tribunal (section 68)
Right to Advocacy	All patients who are subject to compulsion for longer than 72 hours have the right of access to an IMHA section 130A
Young people	16–17 year olds must be treated as adults when considering admission; they must be admitted to an environment suitable to their needs (section 131)
'Bournewood gap' bridged by DOLS safeguards	Amendments to MCA to apply to people who lack capacity for informed consent but where it appears to be in their best interests to protect them from harm to admit them to hospital/care.

Data from Jones (2012)

The Mental Health Acts 1983 and 2007

However, to establish whether the amendments have had a positive impact on user rights, safeguarding, support and enablement opportunities, there needs to be a closer look at some of the changes made by the MHA 2007 (DoH, 2007); the specific areas which will be discussed will be the introduction of Supervised Community Treatment (SCT), patient safeguards such as changes to the use of electroconvulsive therapy (ECT), the introduction of age-appropriate services, advocacy and the revised Code of Practice (DoH, 2007).

Supervised Community Treatment (SCT)/Community treatment: section 17A–section 17G

The Act introduces SCT for patients following a period of detention in hospital; SCTs replace supervised discharges. This allows the Responsible Clinician (RC) to make a SCT for a patient who is detained under section 3 if the relevant criteria have been met and if the Approved Mental Health Professionals (AMHP) agrees that the SCT is a suitable option for a patient. The criteria for making this order are that:

- the patient is suffering from mental disorder of a nature or degree which makes it appropriate for them to receive medical treatment;
- the patient must require medical treatment for their mental disorder for both their own and/or others' safety;

- appropriate medical treatment must be available within the community;
- it is necessary that the RC should be able to exercise the power to recall the patient to hospital.
- and:
- This provision also allows certain conditions to be implemented to ensure that the patient continues to adhere to their treatment plan within the community
- The RC may also recall a community patient to hospital if the patient fails to comply with a condition and if there is a risk of harm to the health or safety of the patient or to other persons if the patient were not recalled to hospital for that purpose (DoH, 2007)

However, Dawson *et al.* (2011) suggest that there appears to be a lack of evidence to support the argument that supervised community treatment orders (CTOs) lead to better treatment outcomes. They make reference to recent research which was undertaken by the Institute of Psychiatry (Churchill *et al.*, 2011), who concluded that:

> *Research in this area has been beset by conceptual, practical and methodological problems, and the general quality of the empirical evidence is poor .... [T]here is currently no robust evidence about either the positive or negative effects of CTOs on key outcomes, including hospital readmission, length of hospital stay, improved medication compliance, or patients' quality of life* (p. 14).

It could be argued that the amendments made to mental health legislation represent the resurgence of the medical model in relation to the broadening of the legal definition of mental disorder, allowing greater medical discretion and the introduction of supervised treatment in the community.

Mental Health Tribunal (MHT)

Amendments have been made by the 2007 Act (DoH, 2007), which has led to the introduction of a power to reduce the time before a case has to be referred to the MHT by hospital managers. Following mounting criticisms and calls for reform within the Tribunal systems, the First-tier Tribunals (Mental Health) (FtTs) were established in 2008 as independent judicial bodies to provide a safeguarding role for people who are subject to the provisions of the MHA. However, despite some improvements appearing to have been made to the review process, there are still some residual difficulties which will continue to impact on the efficacy of the Tribunal structures, such as lack of resources and recent changes to the legal aid system (Butler, 2009).

Age-appropriate services

This provision allows for children under the age of 18 years to be admitted to hospital in an environment which is age appropriate and suitable to meet their needs. There is also a recommendation that specialist child and adolescent services (CAMHS) should be involved, where possible. The Act also confirms that where 16–18-year-olds are deemed to be competent, they have a right to their decisions should be respected, regardless of whether these views differ from those of their parents (Mental Health Alliance, 2009). On the surface, this provision does appear to provide young people more opportunity to exercise their rights to autonomy, however, it should be noted that the High Court still retains its inherent jurisdiction to overrule a young person's decision to refuse treatment (Harbour, 2009).

Electro-convulsive therapy

In Part IV of the Act, various new safeguards have been implemented in the form of consent or second opinions in relation to more controversial or invasive treatments, such as psychosurgery and ECT (section 58A). Where a patient has capacity, a refusal to accept ECT can no longer be overridden, except in life-threatening circumstances. Treatment continuing beyond 3 months also requires a second opinion; any other psychiatric treatment of detained patients may be given compulsorily, in the discretion of the responsible clinician (Fennell, 2011).

Advocacy and rights

The Mental Health Alliance adopted an important role during the development of the new Act primarily in relation to advocating on behalf of the service users and carers for improved outcomes. It was hoped that the amended MHA would provide service users with more positive rights and entitlements. However, Bartlett (2012) suggests that the impact of the MHA 2007 has been to introduce procedures to protect patients whilst detained but still does little to positively promote the cultural, political and economic rights of patients. The Act, as amended does place a duty on relevant authorities to make arrangements for independent mental health advocates (IMHAs) to be made available to all patients who are liable to be detained, including patients who are subject to guardianship and CTOs. The role of the IMHA is to provide support to patients, helping them to understand the statutory powers that they are subject to and how this may be challenged (Brammer, 2010).

However, the Care Quality Commission Annual Report 2010–2011 (CQC, 2011) found that, although there were some examples of good practice within the operation of mental services, one area which required improvement centred around the lack of understanding in relation to the role of IMHAs to support and protect patient rights. The Commission were also concerned that a number of staff still had a limited understanding of the role of the IMHA. Further, in 2012 the Mental Health Alliance and Action for Advocacy suggested that due to a lack of funding, thousands of patients were being denied the right to an IMHA (www.mentalhealthalliance.org.uk/).

Revised Code of Practice and principles

The Code of Practice was originally introduced to provide guidance for doctors, managers and AMHPs in relation to the operation of the Act. The Code of Practice was revised in 2008 (DoH, 2008) following the 2007 Act with the introduction of a statement of guiding principles which include:

- the purpose principle;
- the least restriction principle;
- respect;
- participation;
- effectiveness, efficiency and equity principle.
  (Brayne & Carr, 2012)

Fennell (2011) suggests that although the primary purpose of the Code of Practice (DoH, 2008) is to provide guidance, the principles should be used consistently to promote patient rights and dignity. However, the House of Lords have subsequently ruled that deviation from the Code is permissible if there is 'sufficiently convincing justification'. Despite the commitment to advocacy, guiding principles and rights, Bartlett (2011) suggests that the Act has obscured the reality of medical freedom with the illusion of legal control; 'It is tempting to conclude, on this basis, that the treatment of mental disorder is more about power and control than about beneficence, and that mental health patients are objects in a power play rather than autonomous individuals with rights' (p. 550).

Changes to the Mental Capacity Act 2005

The MHA 2007 has also made amendments to the MCA 2005 (DoH, 2005) by introducing procedures which allow a person in a care or hospital setting, who lacks capacity, to be deprived of their liberty for procedures to authorise the deprivation of liberty of a person resident in a hospital or care home who lacks the capacity to consent. The MCA 2005 provides the authority to detain and treat an incapacitated adult, without consent, with all decisions being made in the person's best interests and in the least restrictive manner. However, it should be noted that the MCA 2005 does not provide authority if the person's treatment is regulated by Part IV of the Act (Fennell, 2011).

The Mental Capacity Act 2005

Introduction

It is a common misconception that the MCA is aimed at people who have a mental health problem; this is not the case. The purpose of the Act is to support users, carers and health/social care professionals who have to deal with someone who may, at present or in the future, lack capacity to make decisions. Therefore, the Act needs to be considered by anyone who cares for someone who lacks capacity, is 16 years or over and lives in England and Wales.

The MCA was passed by Parliament in 2005 and was not implemented until 2007; the purpose of the Act is to provide a statutory framework for decision-making on behalf of people who lack capacity to consent to their care or treatment. It also allows capacitated adults the framework to prepare for a time when they may lack capacity in the future. Before the implementation of the Act, incapacity was usually dealt with under common law doctrine of necessity, which provided care of adults in their 'best interests' (Barber *et al.*, 2012). However, the Act does not prescribe who the decision-maker should be in every instance, although the code of practice does give a mechanism for resolving any disputes in the area.

Five key principles

The Act consists of five key principles to be applied when working with someone who may, at present or in the future, lack capacity:

1) A person must be assumed to have capacity unless it is established that they lack capacity;

The starting point is that there is always a presumption of capacity even after an assessment where this is proven not to be the case. The Act would not expect a formal assessment to be carried out for every day-to-day decision as long as they have reasonable belief that the person lacks capacity and they have an objective reason to believe this to be true.

2) A person is not to be treated as unable to make a decision unless all practicable steps to help them to do so have been taken without success;

When justifying an intervention, the person would have to demonstrate that all reasonable steps have been unsuccessfully made before making a final assessment that a person lacks capacity. The Code of Practice 2.7 gives us some useful guidance regarding the kind of support people might use to help them make a decision, as follows:

- Using different forms of communication (e.g., nonverbal communication);
- Providing information in a more accessible form (e.g., drawings, photographs);
- Treating an underlying medical condition, which may be affecting the persons capacity;
- Having a structured programme to improve a person's capacity to make particular decisions (e.g., develop a new skill that may aid in the decision-making process).

3)   A person is not to be treated as unable to make a decision merely because they make an unwise decision;

Making what others may regard as an unwise decision has been common law in England since 1850; however, the law requires a person to be capable of understanding the consequences of their decision-making. Ashton *et al.* (2006) advise that using this principle, one should consider that there may be circumstances where a person has an ongoing condition which affects their capacity to make a range of sequential decisions. Since one decision on its own makes sense, but when this is combined with other related decisions, it may raise doubts about the person's capacity, or it may prompt a fuller assessment. Nevertheless, importantly, an unwise decision should not by itself, be enough to indicate a lack of capacity.

4)   An act done, or decision made, under the Act for, or on behalf of, a person who lacks capacity must be done, or made, in their best interest;

The principle of best interest has long been established within Common Law, however the Act goes beyond just medical decisions to include social welfare matters. Chapter 5 of the Code of Practice (DoH, 2008) provides a best interest checklist. Brazier and Cave (2007) provide a modified best interest checklist that summarises the main points, as follows:

- In determining best interests, decision-makers should not act merely on the basis of:
   1)   the person's age or appearance;
   2)   a condition or an aspect of their behaviour, which might lead others to make unjustified assumptions about what might be in their best interest.

- In determining best interest, a decision-maker must consider, as far as reasonably possible:

    1) the person's past and present wishes and feelings (and in particular any relevant written statements made by them when they had capacity);
    2) the belief and values that would be likely to influence their decision if they had capacity.

5) Before the act is done, or the decision is made, it should be considered whether the purpose for which it is needed can as effectively be achieved in a way that is less restrictive of the person's rights and freedom of action.

This principle is sometimes referred to as the 'least restrictive alternative'. The important aspect of this principle is to consider whether the purpose for which the decision is needed can be effectively achieved in a less restrictive way. However, the less restrictive way may not be as effective in achieving the purpose, therefore the principle underpinning this is whether any intervention is needed at all and this principle should be considered as part of the decision-making process that consists of all the principles of the Act. This is further supported by the Government document 'No Health Without Mental Health' (DoH, 2012), where the choice, recovery and personalisation agenda is clearly set out for mental health service providers, in that service users' views must be incorporated into clinical practice to secure appropriate support, advice and information regarding their care delivery (Brown *et al.*, 2012; Barber *et al.*, 2012).

Defining mental incapacity

In defining mental incapacity, section 2 of the Act state:

> *A person lacks capacity in relation to a matter if at that material time he is unable to make a decision for themselves in relation to the matter because of an impairment of, or a disturbance in the functioning of, the mind or brain* (DoH, 2005).

Section 3 of the Act provides us with a test that should be used to determine capacity; this is sometimes called the functional test. The section 3 test is that a person is unable to make a decision for themselves if they are unable:

1) to understand the information relevant to the decision;
2) to retain that information;
3) to use or weigh that information as part of the process of making the decision;
4) to communicate their decision (whether by talking, using sign language or any other means).

To further support the health/social care practitioner, it has been proposed that through an implementation of recovery through the organisational change programme, an emphasis on training and education can promote choice, including in a 'crisis' where someone's capacity may be affected. This choice includes the service user's treatment including medication based on best available evidence or a wider range of talking therapies and introduced by Improving Access to Psychological Therapies (IAPT) (DoH, 2012).

Deprivation of liberty under the Mental Capacity Act

Deprivation of Liberty Safeguards (DOLS) (DoH, 2005) were introduced in April 2009 as an amendment to the MCA 2005 as a procedure for the lawful deprivation of liberty of an individual living in a care home or a hospital setting. They apply to someone over the age of 18 years, who lacks capacity and has a mental disorder. As with the MHA, specific criteria need to be met before authorisation of Deprivation of Liberty can be granted. The need for this amendment came from a ruling from the European Court on the implementation of the European Convention on Human Rights regarding a case of the deprivation of liberty of an incapacitated adult. This case is known as *HL versus UK* (2004) or formally known as Bournewood (Barber *et al.*, 2012).

When the European Court of Human Rights reviewed this case, they clearly decided that HL had been deprived of his liberty and awarded damages, as the health care professionals in charge of his care had exercised 'complete and effective control' over his care and movements with a 'degree of intensity' that amounted to a deprivation of liberty. This case only refers up to the first three months until he was detained under the MHA.

The authorisation of Deprivation of Liberty safeguards

If someone is at risk due to incapacity of deprivation of their liberty within a care home or a hospital setting, the DOLS process should be instigated. The managing authority has the responsibility to apply for authorisation of deprivation of liberty. If it is a care home or private hospital, the managing authority will be the person registered under Part 2 of the Care Standards Act 2000 (DoH, 2000b). If it is a NHS hospital, the managing authority is the NHS body responsible for the running of that hospital. Once a 'managing authority' has applied for an authorisation of deprivation of liberty, the 'supervisory body' becomes responsible for consideration of the request. To grant a request, the 'supervisory body' has to commission what is called a 'Six Assessment' (Table 8.2); if all assessment criteria are met, an authorisation of deprivation of liberty can be given. Who may act as a 'supervisory body':

- If the person is receiving treatment in Wales in a hospital, the supervisory body will be the Welsh Minister or a Local Health Board unless a

Table 8.2   The six assessments.

Mental Health	It must be established that the person has a mental disorder as defined in the MHA as amended in 2007. This therefore excludes those with a dependency in alcohol or drugs, but includes those with a learning disability.
Best Interest	It would be in the person's best interest to be detained. It is necessary for the person to be detained to prevent harm to themselves and it is a proportionate response to the likelihood of the person suffering harm and the seriousness of that harm.
Age	The person must be or believed to be 18 years of age or older.
No Refusals	To establish if the authorisation would conflict with any advanced decision-making already made.
Mental Capacity	The capacity of the person must be assessed (as previously described). More detail can be found in sections 1–3 in the MCA (2005)
Eligibility	When assessing eligibility, the assessor must address three questions: Does the patient require treatment for a mental disorder in a hospital? Could the patient be detailed under the MHA (1983)? Is the patient objecting? If all three of these questions are answered positively, a DOLS cannot be authorised and the MHA (1983) must be used.

Data from Brown *et al.*, 2012.

PCT commissions the care and treatment in Wales then they become the supervisory body;

- If a person is in a care home either in England or Wales, the supervisory body will be the local authority for the area that the person normally is a resident of. If the person has no fixed abode, then the supervisory body becomes the local authority where the care home is situated.

The MCA identifies six areas that require an assessment by an appropriate health or social care professional. The six areas identified are: Mental Health, Best Interest, Age, No Refusal, Mental Capacity and Eligibility. For a mental health assessment a doctor approved under section 12 of the 'Mental Health' act or a doctor with a minimum of 3 years postregistration experience in the treatment and diagnosis of mental disorders. For a 'Best Interest' assessment, a qualified AMHP, Social Worker, Nurse Occupational Therapist or Psychologist who has completed approved Best interest Assessment training may be used. The Age and No refusal assessment can be carried out by a Best interest assessor. A 'Mental Capacity' and 'Eligibility' assessment must be carried out by a doctor who is approved as a 'Mental Health' assessor or a

'Best Interest' assessor, but the 'Best interest' assessor for 'Eligibility' assessment must also be an AMHP.

When conducting an assessment, the act gives guidance to the assessor on the criteria for each of the six assessments. In 'Mental Health' it must be established that the person has a mental disorder as defined in the MHA as amended in 2007. This therefore excludes those with a dependency on alcohol or drugs, but includes those with a learning disability. For 'Best Interest', it has to be decided that:

- it would be in the person's best interest to be detained;
- it is necessary for the person to be detained to prevent harm to themselves and that it is a proportionate response to the likelihood of the person suffering harm and the seriousness of that harm.

For 'Age' the person must be or believed to be 18 years of age or older and for 'No Refusals' it would have to be established that any decision that is made does not conflict with any advanced decision-making already made. In the assessment of 'Mental Capacity', the person must be assessed by the principles previously discussed with more details described in section 1–3 of the MCA. Finally, when assessing eligibility, the assessor must address three questions:

- Does the patient require treatment for a mental disorder in a hospital?
- Could the patient be detailed under the MHA (1983)?
- Does the patient object?

If all three of these questions are answered positively a DOLS cannot be authorised and the MHA (1983) must be used.

Urgent authorisation

In an urgent situation, the managing authority can self-authorise for a short period while simultaneously applying for a standard authorisation.

Conclusion

The purpose of the MHA (2007) (DoH, 2007) has been largely to amend existing mental health legislation, to promote service user's and carer's rights whilst also responding to calls for increased supervision within the community. The changes broaden professional roles and responsibilities, introducing a new definition of mental disorder, treatment, and providing age-appropriate services for 16–17 year olds. Independent advocacy services have been developed, and changes to the structure of the Tribunal system aim to promote service user rights more effectively. The Act has also introduced SCT with the aim of preventing repeat readmissions to hospitals through structured community treatment.

Although the changes to mental health legislation have been largely implemented under the rhetoric of increased rights and responsibilities, the uneasy dichotomy between care and control continues to persist. It could be argued that the 2007 reform of the 1983 MHA represents the resurgence of the medical model in relation to the broadening of the legal definition of mental disorder, allowing greater medical discretion and the introduction of supervised treatment in the community. Beresford (2005) suggests that a polarisation exists because of the incompatibility between policies which embrace user involvement and legislation which increases the powers of compulsory treatment and widens the definition of mental disorder.

Despite the fact that current Government policy promotes recovery and service user involvement, ultimately the purpose of the majority of mental health legislation, including the MCA 2005, (DoH, 2005) continues to focus on risk and protection.

The main purpose of the legislation is to ensure that people with serious mental disorders which threaten their health or safety or the safety of the public can be treated irrespective of their consent where it is necessary to prevent them from harming themselves or others (DoH, 2007).

References

Ashton, G., Letts, P., Oates, L. & Terrell, M. (2006) *Mental Capacity: The New Law*. Jordans, London.

Barber, P., Brown, R. & Martin, D. (2012) *Mental Health Law in England and Wales*. Learning Matters, Exeter.

Bartlett, P. (2011) Necessity must be convincingly shown to exist: standards for compulsory treatment for mental disorder under the Mental Health Act 1983. *Medical Law Review*, **19**, 514–547.

Beresford, P. (2005) Social approaches to madness and distress: user perspectives and user know edges. In: *Social Perspectives in Mental Health: Developing Social Models to Understand and Work with Mental Distress* (ed. J. Tew). Jessica Kingsley Publishers, London.

Brammer, A. (2010) *Law for Social Workers*, 3rd edn. Pearson Education Ltd, Harlow.

Brayne, H. & Carr, H. (2012) *Law for Social Workers*, 12th edn. Oxford University Press, Oxford.

Brazier, M. & Cave, E. (2007) *Medicine, Patients and the Law*, 4th edn. Penguin, London.

Brown, R., Barber, P. & Martin, D. (2012) *The Mental Capacity Act 2005: A Guide for Practice*, 2nd edn. Learning Matters, Exeter.

Butler, J. (2009) *Mental Health Tribunals: Law Policy and Procedure*. Jordan Publishing Ltd, Bristol.

Care Quality Commission (CQC) (2011) *Annual Report on the Use of the Mental Health Act; Second Annual Report*. CQC, London.

Churchill, R., Owen, G., Singh, S. & Hotopf, M (2011) *International Experiences of Using Community Treatment Orders*. Institute of Psychiatry, London.

Dawson, J., Burns, T. & Rugkasa, J. (2011) Lawfulness of a randomised trial of the new community treatment order regime for England and Wales. *Medical Law Review*, **19** (1), 1–26.

Department of Health (DoH) (1983) *Mental Health Act 1983: Publications Policy and Guidance*. Office of Public Sector Information, London.

Department of Health (2000a) *Reforming the Mental Health Act: Part 1. The New Legal Framework*. The Stationary Office, London.

Department of Health (2000b) *Care Standards Act*. The Stationery Office, London.

Department of Health (2005) *Mental Capacity Act*. The Stationery Office, London.

Department of Health (2006) *Our Health, Our Care, Our Say*. Office of Public Sector Information, London.

Department of Health (2007) *Explanatory Notes: Mental Health Act 2007*. Office of Public Sector Information, London.

Department of Health (2008) *Code of Practice: Mental Health Act 2007*. The Stationary Office, London.

Department of Health (2011) *No Health without Mental Health: A Cross Government Mental Health Outcomes Strategy for People of All Ages*. Office of Public Sector Information, London.

Department of Health (2012) *No Health without Mental Health: Implementation Framework*. Department of Health, London.

Fennell, P. (2011) *Mental Health Law and Practice*. Jordan Publishing Ltd, Bristol.

Gould, N. & Martin, D. (2012) Mental health law and social work. In: *Social Work with Adults* (ed. M. Davies). Palgrave, Basingstoke.

Harbour, A. (2009) *Children with Mental Disorders and the Law*. Jessica Kingsley Publishers, London.

Jones, R. (2012) *Mental Health Act Manual*, 15th edn. Sweet and Maxwell, London.

Mental Health Alliance (2009) [Online]. Available at http://www.mentalhealthalliance.org.uk/. Accessed on May 6, 2013.

Sainsbury Centre for Mental Health (2007) *Annual Review 2007*. Sainsbury Centre for Mental Health, London.

Chapter 9

Enabling Risk to Aid Recovery

Angela Hall

Teesside University, UK

If you don't risk anything, you might risk everything!

Introduction

This chapter will explore the concept of risk, and positive risk management, in the context of contemporary mental health care planning. The historical and cultural background to risk will be briefly summarised, to aid an understanding in relation to the present dominant attitudes and values that are influencing Mental Health Professionals (MHPs) when trying to help people manage their risks. A recovery approach will be described when trying to measure and predict risk and the need for a collaborative process in order to enable risks to be taken with the aim of promoting the person's journey of recovery. The chapter will conclude with a case example that considers decision-making and risk taking in relation to promoting recovery as part of the care planning process.

Risk can be defined as the probability that negative consequences will follow an action or can be defined as the likelihood that particular adverse events will occur (Woods, 2001). Positive risk management, risk enablement and therapeutic risk taking are all terms that simply involve, weighing the likelihood of a negative consequence against potential therapeutic benefits of a particular behaviour or situation. It is a rational decision made with the potential for either positive or negative outcomes, but which seems worthwhile not only because of the possible benefits, but also because it is believed to be reasonably predictable that the outcome will be positive.

Managing risk situations within mental health care is a particularly complex and challenging issue which can create real dilemmas for the

Care Planning in Mental Health: Promoting Recovery, Second Edition.
Edited by Angela Hall, Michael Wren and Stephan D. Kirby.
© 2013 John Wiley & Sons, Ltd. Published 2013 by John Wiley & Sons, Ltd.

MHP who tries to balance the management of risk with the autonomy and rights of the individual. There is a well-established inquiry culture into standards of mental health care that began in 1632 with the Privy Council Inquiry into conditions at Bethlehem (Bethlam) Hospital (Sheppard, 1995). These have continued over the centuries, initially focusing attention on the care of people within institutions, that is, the 1969 Ely Hospital Inquiry; the Farleigh Hospital Inquiry in 1971; a year later, in 1972, the Whittingham Inquiry; and more recently the care of people within the community such as in 1987, Sharon Campbell and in 1991 Barratt Findley. They both discharged themselves from hospital and went on to stab two separate victims. Three months after these reports, the fatal stabbing of Jonathon Zito by Christopher Clunis occurred (Ritchie *et al.*, 1994). These events and the high-profile media attention they received served to question the safety of a community care policy (DoH, 1990) and to fuel the public fear of people with a mental illness.

We are currently living in a predominantly risk-averse society, where the perception and knowledge regarding risk has advanced considerably due to new technologies, legislation and communication systems. It has in some areas become so nonsensical, such that playing conkers is now banned; throwing a snowball at a stranger is now classed as assault. How has such a situation arisen? It could be answered positively, as an outcome of greater public awareness of personal rights and a greater assertiveness in challenging abuse and neglect particularly in relation to the quality of care received. So it is essential that complaints against public services are effectively investigated, not least because consumer (patient, service user or client) feedback plays a vital role in quality assurance. On the other hand, the compensation culture is facilitated by the fear of costly litigation and the readiness of lawyers to support and vigorously pursue claims.

Safety is a key issue in all areas of society, banking, policing and education as just a few examples, but this is even more so in mental health and it is also more difficult and challenging. 'Patient autonomy has to be considered alongside public safety. A good therapeutic relationship must include both sympathetic support and objective assessment of risk' (DoH, 2007a). The philosophy underpinning the Department of Health, *Best Practice in Risk Management* (DoH, 2007a) framework is one that balances care needs against risk needs, and that emphasises:

- positive risk management;
- collaboration with the service user and others involved in care;
- the importance of recognising and building on the service user's strengths;
- the organisation's role in risk management alongside the individual practitioner's.

(DoH, 2007a)

Risk and regulation

It is not only the fear of litigation that can impact on attitudes to therapeutic risk. Regulation of clinical activity has also markedly increased in recent years. One of the main ways in which risk is managed in any context is through regulation. This is true of society in general, which uses laws and policing to minimise potential harm to its citizens and also of professional bodies such as the General Medical Council, and the Nursing and Midwifery Council which have the power to strike individuals from professional registers if they are found guilty of professional misconduct. It is also true of organisations, which will seek to ensure cost effectiveness by regulating the behaviour and performance of their employees. Organisations that provide public health care are now more intensively regulated than at any time in history, and it is in this context that therapeutic risk must be considered.

Mental health patients have not always been stereotyped as a risk to others. In a mainly rural society, people with mental illness were often accepted and treated charitably (for a history of mental health care, see Roberts, 1981). As the number of people living in cities increased, a large population of urban mentally ill developed. In this environment, they had a greater chance of causing disruption or simply failing to blend in. This led to the building of the early asylums that simply removed the mentally ill from society in the same way that prisons did with criminals. By the eighteenth century, institutions like Bethlehem Hospital (aka Bedlam), were requesting visitors to pay a penny to observe their patients as a form of freak show. This outsider status aroused fear and rejection and a longstanding belief, still evident today, that people with mental health problems are automatically a risk to others.

Along with continuing social prejudice, however, insanity came to be medicalised, seen as a disease to be diagnosed and potentially cured, and in time, although not immediately, the asylums were absorbed into the newly formed National Health Service and became large psychiatric hospitals. These total institutions have in turn given way in recent decades to a wide range of community-based provision, of which inpatient care is now only one aspect. As part of a major public service, mental health care is nowadays subjected to the same kinds of centralised quality control as other public services such as education. This is partly in response to continuing Government drives to ensure standardised, cost-effective health care in response to demands from the electorate. In pursuit of this aim, targets are set and their achievement is monitored by central bodies such as the Healthcare Commission and Care Quality Commission.

Impact of inquiries

National guidance and policy directives have often emerged as a result of major inquiries into mental health care associated with tragedies involving homicide or suicide. One of the most influential was the inquiry into the care and treatment of Christopher Clunis (Ritchie *et al.*, 1994). Christopher Clunis killed Jonathan Zito when he was waiting for a tube train at Finsbury Park. The subsequent inquiry identified a long list of errors and missed opportunities in the care of this patient, stretching back over many years. He had a long history of violence, institutional care and noncompliance with treatment programmes (Ritchie *et al.*, 1994). The inquiry report was particularly scathing in its criticism of the poor coordination between all agencies involved in Christopher Clunis' care despite the introduction of the Care Programme Approach (CPA) in 1991, which was intended to ensure seamless planning and provision of healthcare between services and agencies. The Ritchie Report (1994) led to renewed attempts to operationalise the CPA effectively (DoH, 1994). The main elements of the CPA continue to include:

- systematic arrangements for assessing the health and social needs of people accepted into secondary mental health services;
- the formulation of a care plan which identifies the health and social care required from a variety of providers;
- the appointment of a care coordinator to keep in close touch with the service user and to monitor and coordinate care;
- regular review and, where necessary, agreed changes to the care plan.

Problems in implementing the CPA were addressed in 1999, as part of the Government's reform of mental health services. Case management, the approach to mental health care used by local authorities, was integrated with the CPA into the single system of Care Coordination, featuring:

- a single point of referral;
- a unified health and social care assessment process;
- coordination of the respective roles and responsibilities of each agency in the system;
- access, through a single process, to the support and resources of both health and social care.

(DoH, 1999)

This was further reviewed in 2007 to improve the consistency and reduce the amount of bureaucracy in *Refocusing the Care Programme Approach* (DoH, 2008). There have been many other important inquiries that have influenced attitudes to risk. One such was the Report of the Committee of Inquiry into the events leading up to and surrounding the fatal incident at the Edith Morgan Centre, Torbay, on 1, September 1993 (Blom-Cooper *et al.*, 1995). The incident involved a mental health patient, Andrew Robinson, who stabbed to death an occupational therapist, Georgina Robinson. The inquiry found that:

- The fatal incident was inherently unpredictable;
- For reasons connected with Andrew Robinson's unlawful absence from the Edith Morgan Centre, the homicidal attack was preventable;

- There was a likelihood of some dangerous conduct by Andrew Robinson as a consequence of the removal of a previous Restriction Order by a Mental Health Review Tribunal;
- A previous guardianship application could and should have been renewed;
- There were deficiencies in the mode and manner of communication.

The report also contains a significant chapter on the role of risk assessment and management in care planning. Having shown that the staff in this case had failed to detect Andrew Robinson's risk of violence through their failure to explore his past history, it emphatically states that past behaviour is the best predictor of future behaviour and recommends that the circumstances of any past violence should be rigorously examined.

A further, highly influential example of the inquiry process is provided by the five-yearly *Report of the Confidential Inquiry into Suicide and Homicide by People with Mental Illness, Safety First* (DoH, 2012). Information about every case of suicide or homicide by mental health service users is reported to the confidential inquiry team, which has now compiled an extensive database of evidence and used it to provide recommendations for safe practice in mental health care. Since this is the best evidence available on what makes a safe service, trusts are now audited annually on their compliance with the recommendations of Safety First by the Healthcare Commission.

Among the many standards which must now be met as a result of this inquiry, all mental health staff who work with people at risk must be trained in risk management every 3 years, while, because most suicides have been found to occur in the period after discharge, inpatients who have been at risk must be followed up within 7 days of discharge. The inquiry's previous finding that the main suicidal method is hanging has led to a requirement that likely ligature points in in-patient areas must be removed or covered. This addresses impulsive suicidal acts that make use of immediate suicidal means rather than planned suicides that need to be prevented by effective risk assessment and therapeutic relationships. There has now been a reduction in suicides in inpatient care and the areas now to focus safe practice is within crisis and home-treatment teams (DoH, 2012).

Exploring risk issues

Risk assessment is an essential and ongoing part of the CPA process. Risk assessment, therefore, is about weighing up both the possible beneficial and harmful outcomes of an intervention or procedure and stating the likelihood and extent of either occurring (DoH, 1999).

The ability to measure and predict risk remains a central task for MHPs, however how this is achieved can influence the person's recovery process, it can have a restrictive or inhibiting effect on the person or it can have a reflexive and empowering effect. However, there may be different views between colleagues on how best to enable risk taking (Carpenter *et al.*, 2003) and it is quite common for both health and social work professionals to regard risk to different groups of people, quite differently. For example, in relation to older people, it is often regarded as a threat to their welfare and rarely as an acceptable stimulant or diversion. It is more likely in this context, for service users' choices and behaviours to be seen as leading to dangerous incidents or serious harm (Stevenson, 1999). These views of risk and risk taking, as undesirable and negative, are often influenced by stereotypical and prejudicial views of older people, and should be avoided (Titterton, 2005). Recognising the differences of managing risk for older people, there have been specific guidance (DoH, 2010) developed to enable risk taking, as it was acknowledged that a 'Safety First' approach was disempowering (Clarke *et al.*, 2009; Nuffield Council on Bioethics, 2009) and socially excluding people with dementia (DoH, 2007b). The guidance offers a risk-enabling framework for when risk is an issue for people with dementia (DoH, 2010).

Identifying and predicting risk is not a one-off process, rather it is integral to the ongoing planning of care and must be considered in relation to the person's overall recovery process. It must involve a collaborative exploration of the person's potential to harm and their vulnerability to harm. It is essentially an interpersonal process and often the level of collaboration can be seen as a predictor of risk behaviour. Generally, an effective therapeutic alliance will lead to reduced risk and a poor working alliance is indicative of a higher risk, but of course risk assessment is not an exact science and variations do occur; there is no guarantee, as the chance of risk (harm) occurring is multidimensional and dynamic.

The occurrence of risk behaviour is difficult to prevent but it can be minimised and strategies to improve the quality of a risk assessment are:

- a comprehensive person-focused assessment;
- developing an effective therapeutic alliance;
- encouraging an open and honest debate of issues;
- valuing the person's perspective;
- utilising appropriate assessment tools;
- sharing information to increase collaboration;
- involving the person in taking responsibility for their actions and the possible consequences;
- being aware of the risk situations/behaviours;
- discussing early warning signs and strategies for self-help;
- demonstrating a collaborative approach to care plans/crisis plans.

Sayce (2005) shows how current social care provision is 'utterly permeated by risk-thinking' and how this discriminates against people with mental health problems in particular. Although risk does not always signal danger or urgency, nor necessarily require an emergency response, it may indicate problems, suicidal thoughts and intentions. For example, risky behaviour is often regarded as normal for young men, in contrast to older people, and health and social work professionals might make incorrect assumptions and misinterpret evidence (Oliver & Storey, 2006). Therefore it is imperative that a recovery-focused approach is used to promote the person's quality of life, this can be achieved by recognising the person's natural resilience and strengths (Rapp & Gosha, 2006) when dealing with their vulnerabilities. As problems or risk issues are identified, the person's positive skills should be taken into account as part of the care-planning process. Not only this but the person ideally being responsible in identifying the risk issues they consider to be a priority and how they would prefer any difficult situations to be dealt with, including who are the most appropriate people or services to effectively help them. It is useful to identify any advance decisions that the person may want to happen, in relation to recognising their early warning signs or triggers that may indicate potential risk issues and how these should be planned for.

Enabling risk

The aim of mental health care and treatment is to help restore the person as far as possible to independent functioning. The recovery of independence inevitably involves a degree of risk. However, risk can be reduced as far as possible without compromising the need to allow the person appropriate opportunities to make their own choices and decisions and to act independently. According to the *Best Practice in Managing Risk* framework (DoH, 2007a), 'Positive risk management means being aware that risk can never be completely eliminated, and aware that management plans inevitably have to include decisions that carry some risk' (DoH, 2007a).

Collaboration is an essential aspect of enabling risk and positive risk management. A good relationship based on empathy, warmth and trust are central to enabling an honest and transparent process enabling specific risks to be taken. There may be times, however, when this is not possible due to the nature of the person's mental illness, but it should always be attempted and when people are unable to be involved, the person should be informed of all decisions in an open and honest way.

Positive risk management includes:

- working with the service user to identify what is likely to work;
- paying attention to the views of carers and others around the service user when deciding a plan of action;
- weighing up the potential benefits and harms of choosing one action over another;

- being willing to take a decision that involves an element of risk because the potential positive benefits outweigh the risk;
- being clear to all involved about the potential benefits and the potential risks;
- developing plans and actions that support the positive potentials and priorities stated by the service user, and minimising the risks to the service user or others;
- ensuring that the service user, carer and others who might be affected are fully informed of the decision, the reasons for it and the associated plans;
- using available resources and support to achieve a balance between a focus on achieving the desired outcomes and minimising the potential harmful outcome.

(DoH, 2007a)

If all of these are applied within a collaborative and person-centred approach, then managing risk can be an empowering experience rather than a negative restrictive one. However, it needs to be acknowledged that given the complexion of severe mental illness, there may be times when decisions are based on the immediate threat of danger, it may be at these times that MHPs are required to make decisions for the person in order to protect them or others from potential harm (Ryan, 1999). It may be necessary to utilise the Mental Health Act (1995) due to a person's lack of acknowledgement of the danger or their unwillingness to accept alternative help, even so a collaborative approach to risk management would continue to be the aim, however, distinctive ways of managing this may be required. Some symptoms of mental illness can present the person with a distorted or false reality, thereby preventing their ability to appraise or respond in an appropriate way. It is then reasonable for the MHP to make decisions based on their knowledge of the person and their judgement of what course of action would serve the person best in their recovery (DoH, 2007a). Decisions made about risk management should always involve improving the person's quality of life and their plans for recovery, while remaining aware of the safety needs of the person, their carer and the public (Mersey Care NHS Trust, 2005).

Risk management cycle

Given the context of increased regulation and concerns about complaints and litigation, mental health practitioners face a challenge in seeking to balance the imperatives of safe and defensible care and treatment with the need to avoid paternalistically overprotecting the mental health service user, for whom recovery of functioning can only be achieved by appropriate positive risk-taking. Over-defensive practice is bad practice, yet many MHPs feel in a vulnerable position when dealing with risk, they fear being blamed and open to litigation if harm occurs. There is a dominant culture of 'covering our backs' in many organisations now, and mental health is no exception. However, avoiding all risk is not possible or beneficial for the person in the long run, and can be counterproductive. Imagine if parents prevented children from walking for fear that they may fall and harm themselves, children need to learn to walk and if they fall it is part of the process. While not equating people with mental illness to children, it demonstrates how risks have to be taken in order for people to learn and develop. How can MHPs ensure that they are making the right decision with the person and for the person rather than making themselves feel 'safe'.

When making any risk-related decision, it is likely to be acceptable if:

- it conforms with relevant guidelines;
- it is based on the best information available;
- it is documented;
- the relevant people are informed.

(DoH, 2007a)

As long as a decision is based on the best evidence, information and clinical judgement available, it will be considered defensible, if harm were to occur to anyone. Defensible practice, proceeding responsibly on the basis of evidence, is not defensive practice, aimed at avoiding harm at the expense of the person's recovery of independence, which would be the opposite of therapeutic. MHP can achieve this balance by approaching therapeutic risk systematically (Table 9.1). The process can be seen as a simple and logical cycle.

Table 9.1 Systematic risk identification.

Identify the potential for risk	Mental health service users are at risk not just for suicide or self-harm but also for violence, self-neglect, abuse and other kinds of harm. Each person must be approached as an individual who may face a particular and fluctuating range of risks in different circumstances.
Assess the risk	Risk assessment is not an exact science. While a wide range of risk assessment tools have been produced and published, in themselves they will yield too many false positives (i.e., predict too many people to be at risk who are not) and so are more of a help rather than an alternative to subjective decision-making. However, risk assessment should always be approached systematically to ensure that all potential risk factors are considered. Both actuarial risk factors, such as social group, gender or age, and clinical risk factors related to the person's mental health problem, past history and mood need to be included in any comprehensive risk assessment.
Rate the risk	Quantitative risk-assessment tools do exist in mental health and are identified as best practice. More usually, however, risk assessment is descriptive and levels of

Table 9.1 (*Continued*)

	risk may be expressed as being high, medium, or low. If this is so, it is essential that understanding of the meaning of these adjectives is shared among a clinical team, since subjective interpretations of particular words vary widely and there is a danger of misunderstanding.
Take preventive action	Action plans to address risk need to be integrated with the rest of the person's care, and for mental health service users should come within the standards of the CPA. The Care Plan should be coordinated and monitored by a single coordinator and it should be shared with the service user. This is the stage where the balance between care and control can be responsibly addressed. Preventive actions need to be considered in the context of therapeutic actions: for example, a period of home leave may seem to be essential for the person's recovery, but at the same time a risk may well be involved in allowing the person to spend time away from the clinical setting.
Evaluate the success of preventive action	Risk-management measures must be continuously monitored for effectiveness and if they are not effective must be changed.
Revisit the potential for risk	The risk-management cycle always needs to return to its beginning. Risks vary and fluctuate, one risk may be replaced with another, or risks may have been permanently reduced.

Data from Doyle, 1999

Many of the factors involved in predicting and measuring risk and enabling risk as part of positive risk management which have been discussed in this chapter can be illustrated using a Case Example 9.1:

Case Example 9.1 Peter: enabling risk to promote recovery.

Peter has a 2 year history of severe depression. He has a past history of self-harm, including two suicide attempts, involving trying to throw himself in front of a car (2 years ago) and apparently trying to hang himself (a year ago), although on this occasion he did so when he could be interrupted by his wife.

Peter has now been on the ward for 3 months. He is detained under section 3 of the Mental Health Act (1983). He has been under varying levels of observation during that time, including several periods of constant observation to prevent him harming himself and several periods of intermittent observation. He continues to say that his life has no meaning, that he is a burden to everyone and that he should be allowed to kill himself. As he has been relatively stable in recent days, staff have been trying to take therapeutic risks by allowing him unescorted time off the ward but not out of the building in order to go to occupational therapy sessions. Yesterday the nurse in charge, with the agreement of the responsible medical officer, allowed Peter to go for a short walk on his own in the grounds. Although there is a busy road nearby, he returned at the agreed time with no apparent problems and reported having enjoyed the fresh air.

On arriving on duty today Peter asks the nursing staff if he can have another walk on his own. He appears to be relatively calm in mood.

Discussion:

In terms of the risk-management cycle:

1. There is a potential risk to Peter: he has a number of risk factors for self-harm and suicide and past behaviour is an important predictor for future behaviour. The risk is immediate and has the potential to be fatal;
2. From the information available, the risk appears to be medium. However, his calm mood may be assumed in order to secure an opportunity to leave the ward, or he may genuinely be feeling calm because he intends to end his problems soon by taking his own life;
3. Preventive options available include refusing leave, allowing escorted leave only or seeking further assessment before making a decision;
4. Involving Peter in the decision-making process is essential to give him choice and responsibility while empowering him in his recovery;
5. Whatever decision is made, the decision must be evaluated. At some stage, Peter will have to be allowed leave and a full record must be made of what happened to inform his future care;
6. The multidisciplinary team should discuss the issue and plans made for the next time Peter asks for leave.

In order to recover independent functioning, Peter needs to be allowed graduated periods of autonomy. He could be protected from self-harm to a large extent by being obliged to remain on the ward, but this would be at the cost of his confidence and it is likely that it would become increasingly stressful for him. MHPs have a duty to try to promote Peter's recovery of independence while at the same time ensuring that the risks to him are minimised. As a self-determining individual, it is possible that Peter could use a period of leave to harm himself, for example by hanging or throwing himself in front of a car as he has in the past. If he did, the staff could claim that they were acting in his best interests and that any reasonable body of mental health practitioners would have acted as they did. However, in order to justify their claim, the staff would need to demonstrate that, like any reasonable body of practitioners, they had tried to minimise the risks inherent in allowing him a period of leave. They could do this firstly by ensuring that the decision to allow him leave complied with the terms of the Mental Health Act: as Peter was a detained patient, the responsible medical officer would have to sign a section 17 form (DoH, 1983) specifying the conditions of his leave. There may be other Trust policies that would need to be considered. Further, the staff should carry out and record an individual risk assessment, since risks fluctuate and they could not rely only on his behaviour the previous day or on the actions of other staff. It would be essential that the staff member who made this assessment had up-to-date training in risk management. Finally, in terms of managing the risk, staff have the option of refusing leave (with an explanation to Peter), of agreeing to leave with an escort, or of allowing unescorted leave. In the end, a decision has to be made, and it is possible that the decision could have tragic consequences. Nonetheless, the staff are acting responsibly and in Peter's interests if they enable risk taking which they can demonstrate was justified.

Staff

Mental health staff themselves can reduce therapeutic risk by ensuring that their own practice is of an optimum standard. Service users have a right to expect that the risks involved in their care and treatment are minimised by the fact that they are in the hands of staff who are skilled and knowledgeable in their field. It is reasonable for them to expect that staff receive clinical supervision rather than practising in a vacuum; that they are continually developing as professionals through appraisal and learning; that their practice is supported by evidence, via clinical guidelines and protocols; that they communicate effectively with each other and record their actions and observations; that they will involve service users themselves as far as possible in their own care and that they take note of and learn from adverse incidents.

Systems

Effective multidisciplinary and multiagency working is essential if risks are to be minimised. Team development can be used to promote effective communication and decision making that makes best use of the varied skills, knowledge and experience of the different team members. This was a lesson that the Georgina Robinson Inquiry Report (Blom-Cooper *et al.*, 1995) drew: had information from all the professionals in the team involved been heeded, the tragic outcome might have been avoided. If the CPA is to be used effectively to minimise risk, it is essential that involvement and communication between mental health workers and primary care workers such as the GP, together with other agencies such as housing and the police, is a reality rather than a paper exercise.

Conclusion

As this chapter has shown, despite the pressures of potential litigation and the demands of national guidance and regulations, it is always in the interests of the wellbeing and recovery of the person that appropriate therapeutic risks are not compromised by defensive practice. By approaching care and treatment systematically, with an awareness of legal, professional and policy requirements and through constantly maintaining their own professional competencies, MHPs can ensure that care planning across professional and organisational boundaries has the potential to be both therapeutically effective and – not defensive but *defensible*.

Acknowledgement

The editors wish to acknowledge Dr David Duffy (retired) for his original chapter in the first edition of this text which formed the basis for this current chapter.

References

Blom-Cooper, L., Hally, H. & Murphy, E. (1995) *The Falling Shadow: One Patient's Mental Health Care 1978–1993*. Duckworth, London.

Carpenter, J., Schneider, J., Brandon, T. & Wooff, D. (2003) Working in multidisciplinary community mental health teams: the impact on social workers and health professionals of integrated mental health care. *British Journal of Social Work*, **33** (8), 1081–1103.

Department of Health (DoH) (1983) *The Mental Health Act 1983*. HMSO, London.

Department of Health (1990) *National Health Service and Community Care Act*. HMSO, London.

Department of Health (1994) *Implementing Care for People: Care Management*. HMSO, London.

Department of Health (1999) *Effective Care Coordination in Mental Health Services:· Modernising the Care Programme Approach, a Policy Booklet*. The Stationery Office, London.

Department of Health (2007a) *Best Practice in Managing Risk; Principles and Evidence for Best Practice in the Assessment and Management of Risk to Self and Others in Mental Health Services*, DoH, London.

Department of Health (2007b) *Putting People First: A Shared Vision and Commitment to the Transformation of Adult Social Care*, DoH, London.

Department of Health (2008) *Refocusing the Care Programme Approach: Policy and Positive Practice Guidance*, DoH, London.

Department of Health (2010) *Equality Act*, DoH, London.

Department of Health (2012) *Safety First: Five-Year Report of the National Confidential Inquiry into Suicide and Homicide by People with Mental Illness*. The Stationery Office, London.

Doyle, M. (1999) Organisational responses to crisis and risk: issues and implications for mental health nurses. In: *Managing Risk in Mental Health Nursing* (ed. T. Ryan). pp. 40–56. Stanley Thornes, London.

Mersey Care NHS Trust (2005) *Policy and Procedures for the use of Clinical Risk Assessment Tools, Policy no. SA10*. Mersey Care NHS Trust, Liverpool.

Oliver, C. & Storey, P. (2006) *Evaluation of Mental Health Promotion Pilots to reduce Suicide amongst Young Men: Final Report*. Thomas Coram Research Institute, London.

Rapp, C.A. & Goscha, R.J. (2006) *The Strengths Model: Case Management with People with Psychiatric Disabilities*. Oxford University Press, Oxford.

Ritchie, J., Dick, D. & Lingham, R. (1994) *The Report of the InquiryiInto the Care and Treatment of Christopher Clunis*, HMSO, London.

Roberts, A. (1981) *Mental Health History Timeline*, [Online]. Available at http://www.flutrackers.com/forum/showthread.php?t=13016. Accessed on .

Ryan, T. (1999) *Managing Crisis and Risk in Mental Health Nursing*. Stanley Thornes, London.

Sayce, L. (2005) Risks, rights and anti-discrimination work in mental health: avoiding the risks in considering risk. In: *Social Work Futures: Crossing Boundaries, Transforming Practice* (eds R. Adams, L. Dominelli & M. Payne). pp. 167–181. Palgrave Macmillan, Basingstoke.

Sheppard, D. (1995) Learning the lessons. In: *Managing Risk in Mental Health Nursing* (ed. T. Ryan). Stanley Thornes, London.

Stevenson, O. (1999) Old people at risk. In: *Risk Assessment in Social Care and Social Work* (ed. P. Parsloe). pp. 201–216. Jessica Kingsley Publishers, London.

Titterton, M. (2005) *Risk and Risk Taking in Health and Social Welfare*. Jessica Kingsley Publishers, London.

Woods, P. (2001) Risk assessment and management. In: *Forensic Mental Health Practice: Issues in Practice* (eds C. Dale, T. Thompson, & P. Woods), pp. 85–98. Baillière Tindall, London.

Chapter 10

Collaborating Across the Boundaries

Mike Wren, Stephan D. Kirby and Angela Hall

Teesside University, UK

Introduction

This chapter will explore the core features that are vital for any professional who is involved in the life of the person with mental health needs, and those closest to them, to proactively encourage collaboration. We need to acknowledge that collaboration with others must be consistently applied in terms of the roles, responsibilities and human resource capabilities working across their multiprofessional boundaries for them to be effective and for the ultimate benefit of the person. It is widely known that mental health problems are a common feature of our society where one in four people will experience mental health problems at some point in their lives. Many of the causes of mental health problems are socially determined, and so many of the changes that can lead to better mental wellbeing and recovery lie within the person's own wider social environment. The importance of collaboration cannot, therefore, be underestimated especially when you also consider that nine out of ten people affected by mental health problems report having experienced stigma and discrimination. For example, from within their own family and friendship networks, and typically when striving to gain meaningful employment, as well as in public services such as health, welfare and justice. Such costs, when translated into the current austere economics and not investing in the effective so-called joining up of mental health provisions, are clear and equate to mental ill health costing over £105 billion every year (DoH, 2005a).

The chapter will equally establish transferable approaches that can both respond to and can (in some part) positively enhance the clarion cry for a continued rejuvenation of the safe, effective and efficient deployment of recovery-oriented, prevention, community-based and person-focused inter-relationships to coexist between a variety of collaborative roles, relationships

Care Planning in Mental Health: Promoting Recovery, Second Edition.
Edited by Angela Hall, Michael Wren and Stephan D. Kirby.
© 2013 John Wiley & Sons, Ltd. Published 2013 by John Wiley & Sons, Ltd.

and resources working together for the benefit of the person experiencing mental distress and those closest to them. It will also explore the influences, philosophies and reputable approaches that can be adopted to enhance and sustain such collaborative interactions. Also introduced will be the relevant policy drivers that underpin their implementation that influences the future, collective, promotion of mental wellbeing and recovery with genuine attempts for 'collegiate collaboration' to be transcended across as broad a range of boundaries as possible within contemporary mental health practice.

Collaborative roles, responsibilities and resources

The delegation of collaborative roles, responsibilities and resources in our experience is an integral feature of communities of interests to challenge silo thinking and segregation of actions that still continue to prevail. Such concerted efforts include a multitude of organisations, individuals and governmental departments that will, and indeed should, have many different (and at times conflicting) perspectives, viewpoints and motives. These are all essential for building the debate to achieve a robust mental health strategy in the UK, where in the future, the vital human, physical and financial resources are more explicitly, as well as generically, cascaded. This would be inherent within the promotion of proactive engagement and involvement of those whose lives, and those closest to them, have been affected by mental ill health. However, we also acknowledge that these diverse interactions of involved engagement must also have due regard to what we refer to (for the purposes of this chapter) as 'collaborative responsibilities' that include the following:

Renewing our collective commitment to early intervention and recovery-oriented approaches: Anyone who is passionate about maintaining a recovery-oriented approach towards forging meaningful relationships, gainful employment and cocreating wider livelihood networks is much more likely to be able to offer the earliest possible help, advice and support to people experiencing mental distress and those closest to them. This is achieved by utilising opportunities to tap into the knowledge, skills and experiences of the person, and a myriad of other people, to establish the support that is articulated from the person themselves as being of most benefit to them.

Reclaiming relationship-based approaches: It is essential that we cocreate a sense of coherent commonalities that are applicable to a wider population. These would need to be an increased need and a sense of urgency to ensure (by as many means as possible) that collaborative and coordinated approaches are widely disseminated across public, not for profit, and community-based alliances. This would achieve reciprocal resilience, especially in times of increased stress and by channelling specific support for people at the highest risk of experiencing mental ill health throughout their lives.

Tackling inequality: Within our diverse, multicultural and multispiritual societies, there are wide inequalities in the delivery of, take up, and access to mental health communities of support. Community engagement, peer groups, user and carers alliances have predominantly led the way for many years in ensuring that mental health services have, at the heart of their coexistence, the primary aim of helping people get back to the lives they want for themselves. This is achieved through offering assistance, enablement and support to people of all ages and backgrounds to achieve their personal recovery goals, however long it takes.

This includes those livelihood networks that can both contribute to recovery or relapse, and vice versa, and require the establishment of some sensitive brokerage between identifying appropriate accommodation, employment, education, meaningful relationships and financial considerations. This would have entitlement as its focus, rather than dependency and build whatever matters and that can contribute to the stability of the personal life of the person and those closest to them.

Consolidating collaborative values and principles: There continues to be considerable debate about a coherent set of values and principles that could underpin collaborative, interprofessional working environments. This is not to say that any one profession can hold an exclusive claim over others. Rather that their interactions consistently convey a predominantly value-based practice approach, one that is more about combining values and core beliefs that could well be differently expressed according to the roles and responsibilities assigned to the respective professionals that are engaged in interprofessional working or educational arrangements and opportunities (CAIPE, 1997; Braye & Preston-Shoot, 2001; Quinney, 2006; SCIE, 2012).

Clark (2000) identifies eight rules (taken from within generic social work practices) that are features for replicating good practice. They are also written with four guiding ethical principles that (when combined together with other approaches) are potentially transferable as we strive to develop a collegiate set of collaborative working principles. Those transcend mental health care professional boundaries must also be taken into consideration the care-v-control ethical dilemmas, which continue to confront all professions committed to upholding the worth and uniqueness of the person, their entitlement to justice, aspirations of freedom and the essentiality of community presence to encourage recovery. These eight 'rules' consist of 'respectfulness', 'honesty and truthfulness', 'being knowledgeable and skilful', 'being careful and diligent', 'being effective and helpful', 'ensuring also that your work is legitimate and authorised', 'collaborative and accountable' and 'reputable and creditable' (Clark, 2000).

These 'rules' appear compatible to collaborative mental health practice, wherever it exists, and although this is biased predominantly towards community-based networks of support, it is also applicable wherever hospitalisation or rehospitalisation is the only recourse available after all alternatives have been exhausted in the best interests of the person, public and society. It is important, therefore, to consider other reputable approaches to guide what can be potentially contentious, conflicting and contradictory practice. Yet these must continue to remain person-centred and recovery oriented within individual, as well as collective, practices. They must be genuinely offered in a bid to maintain the respective identity of the various professionals involved. There needs to be the continued drive to foster the collective maintenance of an innovative vision; one that continually seeks to enhance collaborative communities of engagement, which are capable of translating a series of comparable and wherever possible collective capabilities.

This vision reaffirms the importance of synergy between the personal qualities and values that are deemed to be essential for strengthening the basis of developing any effective collaborative, alliance-based relationships (as discussed in Chapters 5 and 11) with people experiencing mental health problems and those closest to them. It is not a recent discovery that there are correlations between the importance of therapeutic relationships (alliances) and the positive effect this has on that therapy. The link between personal and professional qualities and developmental opportunities is equally important in relation to the enhancement of a mental health professional's performance when working across the professional boundaries of mental health and social care environments. These interrelated themes suggest a set of generic qualities that demand a considerable degree of sensitivity, knowledge and expertise and for professionals to be self-aware, approachable, purposeful, flexible, reflective and ordinary.

To further support this generic approach to specialised aspects of practice, and to establish the formation of effective mental health care of the future, the adoption of a collective trans-professional value base is essential; one that has currency in direct response to the need for collaborative alliance-based therapeutic relationships. Williams and Dale (2001) identified six specific professional value-based perspectives applicable to, and that should be inherent across, all aspects of mental health and social care namely:

Value 1: Respect the person as a human being, regardless of behaviour, diagnosis or any offending profile;

Value 2: Acceptance and application of current concepts of mental disorders and need for care and treatment operated by the medical, mental health and social care professions;

Value 3: Not judging people;

Value 4: Applying an equally high quality of care to every person;

Value 5: Treating all people with equality and fairness;

Value 6: Maintaining confidentiality.

The interrelationship between the mutual understanding of the multiplicity of roles, responsibilities and resources, as well as the development of a lexicon of collective expressions, will require a significant change to break out of the largely accepted way of single silo working, which is a jargon laden and segregated, centralised structure. It is obvious that we need to engender an ethos that is truly empowering that features a mutually dynamic relationship that is defined by a collegiate acceptance that

- Mental health care is a developmental human activity concerned with helping people live through or to overcome distress;
- The relationship, which is the prism for the therapeutic alliance, is focused upon helping people to reauthor their lives, by confronting and healing past distress, through the alleviation of present distress and thus opening ways to further development;
- Mental health care is focused upon everyday life, the people and their relationship with themselves and others within the context of their interpersonal world;
- Mental health care involves the process of mutual influence; the people with the mental health problems influence the professionals who in turn influence the people and so on. Health care is done *with* people not *to* them. It should be remembered that all mental health care professionals cannot empower people with mental problems; rather, the person empowers the professionals.

(Barker, 1990)

This proactive approach to the conjoining of people experiencing mental health problems, those closest to them and the professionals seeking to work alongside them are each succinctly summarised within many aspects of the *Ten Essential Shared Capabilities* (DoH, 2005b). These, we feel, encompass themes of mutual collegiate interest that rely upon all of us developing together; sharing and interlinking skills, knowledge(s) and experiences. Initially, this could be achieved by a commitment to more interprofessional educational opportunities being made widely available and accessible.

We need to ensure that we continue to collaboratively advocate for, and are reliably informed by, the sharing of the mutual benefits to be gained for all involved in continuing to proactively promote recovering interdependent functioning via the consistent application of opportunities for

Working in partnership: Developing and maintaining constructive working relationships with people with mental health problems, carers, families, colleagues, lay people and wider community networks. Working positively with any tensions created by any, and all, conflicts of interests or aspiration that may arise between the partners in care.

Respecting diversity: Working in partnership with people with mental health problems, carers, families and colleagues to provide care and interventions that not only make a positive difference but also do so in many ways that respect and value diversity including age, race, culture, disability, gender, spirituality and sexuality.

Practising ethically: Recognising the rights and aspirations of people with mental health problems and their families, acknowledging any, and all, power differentials and minimising them whenever possible. Providing treatment and care that is accountable to people with mental health problems and carers within the boundaries prescribed by national, professional, legal and local codes of ethical practice.

Challenging inequality: Addressing the causes and consequences of stigma, discrimination, social inequality and exclusion on people with mental health problems, carers and mental health services. Creating, developing or maintaining valued social roles for people in the communities they come from.

Promoting recovery: Working in partnership to provide care and treatment that enables people with mental health problems and carers to tackle mental health problems with hope and optimism and to work towards a valued lifestyle within, and beyond, the bounds of their mental health problem.

Identifying people's needs and strengths: Working in partnership to gather information to agree health and social care needs in the context of the preferred lifestyle and aspirations of people with mental health problems, their families, carers and friends.

Providing service user-centred care: Negotiating achievable and meaningful goals, primarily from the perspective of people with mental health problems and their families. Influencing and seeking the means to achieve these goals and clarifying the responsibilities of the people who will provide any help that is needed, including systematically evaluating outcomes and achievements.

Making a difference: Facilitating access to, and delivering, the best quality, evidence-based, value-based health and social care interventions to meet the needs and aspirations of people with mental health problems, their families and carers.

Promoting safety and positive risk taking: Empowering the person with mental health problems to decide the level of risk they are prepared to take within health and safety parameters. This includes working with the tension between promoting safety and positive risk taking, including assessing and dealing with possible risks for people with mental health problems, carers, family members and the wider public.

Personal development and learning: Keeping up to date with changes in practice and participating in lifelong learning, personal and professional development for one's self and colleagues through supervision, appraisal and reflective practice (DoH, 2005b).

We acknowledge that exposure alone to a learning environment or opportunities does not equate to enhancing interprofessional education; where two or more professionals learn from, and about, each other to develop their skills and knowledge for collaboration and to improve the quality of care (CAIPE, 1997). The development of delivering more effective collaborative working arrangements and services into future practice is further highlighted in Chapter 13 and by Barr (2002) and Quinney (2006) who acknowledge the complexity of establishing such collaborative educational interrelationships, which require a broader exploration and understanding of what effective learning for collaborative practice might consist of and how this can be supported and achieved. They recommend that for interprofessional education to be effective in the longer term, it must put people with mental health problems at the centre of all activity. It must promote collaboration by reconciling competing professional or agency objectives to reinforce the collaborative competencies/capabilities being demonstrated across professional boundaries thereby driving collaboration in learning and practice to a coherent rationale. Further incorporation of interprofessional values that are common and comparative to learning and employing a range of interactive learning methods, can be counted towards qualification. This supports the need for interprofessional education programmes, and the inclusion of participant experiences, to be evaluated and their findings widely disseminated (Barr, 2002).

In our pursuit to cocreate advantageous, collegiate, collaboration across professional boundaries, we must surely be willing to confront the challenges that often stem from constructs built from within the boundaries of our own professions. Once these have been identified, we can then explore the many advantages that can contribute to a more optimistic and holistic approach towards enhancing collaborative relationships that sustain interprofessional learning and shared working opportunities as an integral feature across interprofessional education, training and curriculum developments of the future.

Collaborating across professional boundaries

What helps and hinders?

Meads *et al.* (2003) suggest that the multiplicity of differences between professionals, organisations or teams could be viewed as a source of continual conflict caused by professionals feeling marginalised and behaving in a defensive way in response to restrained resources. While other groups could equally view this as an opportunity to cocreate sources of creativity as well as innovations in practice to actually transform interprofessional working, thinking and behaviour. Barrett and Keeping (2005) developed creative inter-professional working concepts and offered the following features. Not as a prescriptive framework to be slavishly followed, but rather to provide oppor-tunities for collaborative, collegiate communities of the future to work together, in an holistic way, so as to enhance or harmonise interprofessional practices particularly when collaborating across professional boundaries.

Knowledge of professional roles: It is important to be aware of the roles and responsibilities of other professionals as well as having a clear understand-ing of your own role;

Willing participation: The motivation and commitment for collaborative prac-tice are important if it is to be achieved along with expectations that are realistic and a positive belief in their potential effectiveness;

Confidence: This refers to personal and professional confidence being achieved through experience and built upon a clear professional identity and an understanding of, and belief in, the particular role that the individual pro-fession involved in mental health care can contribute;

Open and honest communications: This includes active listening and con-structive feedback that seeks to clarify and develop understanding;

Trust and mutual respect: This takes time to develop and is essential for people to feel 'safe' to be able to deal with areas that are challenging or that may lead to conflict;

Power: The adoption of a nonhierarchical structure where power is shared is the preferred model, but responsibility and accountability need to be made clear. Power sharing can be difficult to negotiate and is complicated by power being located and experienced at personal, professional and societal levels;

Aspects of conflict: These can be minimised by the application of clear ground rules and a reflective and open approach, and in doing so it will help prevent and resolve conflict. However, conflict can also produce creativity and energy too!

Support and commitment at a senior level: Change and support at all levels is a prerequisite for effective collaborative working;

Professional culture: Language, traditions, ideologies or perspectives asso-ciated with different, individual, insular and professional groups may hinder collaborative working; but also provide the opportunity for new viewpoints to be considered;

Uncertainty: About roles, boundaries and future development need to be acknowledged and addressed;

Envy: Tensions can arise from professional envy and rivalry (territorialism or agency preciousness) created between individuals and organisations, especially when competing for diminishing resources and maintaining power;

Defences against anxiety: Working alongside people with complex problems and within complex structures can create anxiety that can become displaced onto other team members (Barrett & Keeping, 2005).

Despite compelling evidence to the contrary, the public enquiries into the failures of deploying effective communication, efficient collaboration and the skilful coordination of professional and public service efforts to promote the safeguarding of vulnerability, mental, financial, medical and social wellbeing have continued to have a consistent hampering impact upon encouraging collective working arrangements that are specifically targeted towards fostering appropriate professional relationships from within mental health services.

This has led to the difficult fact, and acknowledgement, that undoubtedly these failures (across all professional groups and organisations) have had dire and tragic consequences for individuals and with some stark lessons needing to be learnt about how best to harness skills, knowledge(s) and experience(s) across the professionals and professional groups charged with acting in the best interests of the individual, their family and the protection of the wider public in society (Laming, 2003; SCIE, 2012). We acknowledge that there is no single or correct model, framework or approach for developing collaboration in practice. However, our starting point for this is by accepting that there are a range of good practices (e.g., Multi-Agency Public Protection Agency (MAPPA); *No Secrets* (DoH, 2000); Protection of Vulnerable Adults (POVA)) that strive to safeguard the welfare of vulnerable people. These models demand us to utilise aspects of legal or policy requirements to engage collaborative working opportunities that can be consistently formed via therapeutic alliances and closer consideration of relation-based approaches within contemporary mental health and social care practices. We seek to motivate you (the reader) to be informed by the very people who are experiencing mental health problems and those closest to them working together to actively pursue engagement with a variety of community allies. This can only be achieved effectively by tapping into a combination of experiences, skills and capabilities being appraised alongside the research as well as government claims about the effectiveness (or otherwise) of current collaborative working arrangements in order to realistically inform future development, enhancement and most importantly coherent implementation.

Policy drivers

Principles and philosophies to promote collegiate collaboration

The concept of creating collegiate, collaborative, partnerships in mental health care is not a new phenomenon, indeed from at least the enactment of the original Mental Health Act (DoHSS, 1959), and transcending into contemporary practice, there are many examples of various models of collaborative working. These have continued to be developed and based upon on a growing recognition that no single profession has a monopoly on the necessary skill(s), knowledge(s) and expertise in dealing with the physical, social and psychological difficulties confronting people with mental health needs and those closest to them. However, it is important to consider from the outset of our collaborative journey towards promoting recovery of interdependent functioning the difference between policy-based evidence and evidence-based policy, and their consequential impact upon collaborative, interprofessional education and practice. Policy-based evidence is utilised to support or justify a policy retrospectively, and evidence-based policy is adopted to inform the development of policy (Barrett & Keeping, 2005; Quinney, 2006).

Hudson (2002) refers to these policies or political approaches as the 'interprofessionality' of health and social care and explores 'pessimistic' versus 'optimistic' models of interprofessional and collaborative relationships in practice. He described a 'pessimistic' model of interprofessional working with the sceptical view of whether it is possible to initiate effective collaborative practice between different professional groups.

Collaborative interprofessional working arrangements across boundaries are even more complicated in light of the current coalition government approaches towards modernising public services. The reality is that colleagues who represent interprofessional teams and organisations operate on a series of multiple interchanges taking place between differing perspectives drawn from the individual, organisational, team and professional group levels using their discretion and judgement, which can often contribute to increased conflict and tensions on the effectiveness (or otherwise) of forging collaborative working communities with other colleagues and their respective professions. Issues of professional identity, status, discretion and accountability are influential considerations when striving to deliver effective collaborative working opportunities between different professional groups.

While a strong professional identity for a social worker, nurse or occupational therapist, for example, may well be seen as important, it also has been found that this can create barriers to collaborative working when the different professionals do not share the same beliefs about the valuable contributions that each can bring to the team. This may be expressed as conflicts over beliefs about the perception of services being universal or means tested/targeted. There remains a lack of clarity about team roles, particularly where knowledge and skills over-lap, alongside misunderstandings about the relative merits of medical-v-social models, polarisations of approaches based on deficits, strengths and concerns about constrained discretion with increased accountability.

Hudson's (2002) 'optimistic' view is based on three reasons to support the promotion of interprofessionality across professional boundaries:

Normative reasons: This suggests that interprofessionality is a good thing, and the need to develop closer working is a normal feature of organisations, especially in a climate of increasing demands and limited resources;

Policy reasons: This emphasises that the approach is policy driven in health and social care settings (and associated services), and it has a growing momentum and seems to incorporate a view that interprofessional ways of working are inevitable;

Academic reasons: This demonstrates that given the inevitability of needing to work interprofessionally, academics are challenged to make a 'more construc-tive' contribution to the policy debates by testing out a positive hypothesis (Hornby & Atkinson, 2000; Hudson, 2002; Quinney, 2006).

A series of government documents: *The Mental Health Act* (DoH, 1983, 2007); *Care Programme Approach* (DoH, 1997); *The Mental Capacity Act* (DoH, 2005) and *Think Family* (SCIE, 2012) highlight and promote the importance of effective interprofessional education, working and collaboration in an attempt to ensure the future delivery of high-quality care by enhancing col-laboration with the person with mental health problems and their commu-nity networks. These aspects of policy are significantly evident within the development and subsequent implementation of the *National Service Framework for Mental Health* (DoH, 1999). Its overarching aim provided long-term strategies for improving particular areas of health and social care by actively connecting involvement with initiatives that ranged from coronary heart disease, cancer care, diabetes and long-term conditions to working within older people, mental health care (based upon earlier interventions) that were underpinned often with a community-based, prevention and per-son-centred focus. A key policy driver of this approach, with regards to men-tal health in particular, was the requirement that all those involved in developing this framework do so in consultation with people with mental health problems and carers as well as a wide range of health and social care professionals. This went across many partner agencies whose primary roles were to minimise the impact of a medical condition by working in collaboration with others. This interagency working demonstrated outcomes that were based upon effective partnership working opportunities, alongside direct work with people experiencing mental health problems and those closest to them.

The emergence of Clinical Commissioning Groups was formally convened from April 2012 in response to the enactment of the *Health & Social Care Act* (DoH, 2011) and is the current (coalition) government's approach to improve local health care. By working collaboratively with community-based professionals, public services and the wider general public, it is hoped to avoid duplication of service delivery and ensure value for money by sharing acute, community and mental health provisions that remain localised and to maintain effective engagement through locality meetings and offer some potential opportunities for synergy and the sharing of good practice across professional boundaries. The vision being to collectively tackle health inequalities related to life expectancy, deprivation and poverty indicators across the configurations of previous localities of Primary Care Groups (PCGs) and encapsulating General Practioners (GPs) as commissioners alongside local authorities, public health, facilitation and public protection agency developments each collaboratively responding to (local) targets and initiatives as opposed to national ones.

A common set of values that relate to this new reconfiguration of patient-centred services is based upon supporting continuous improvements mapped to respect; honesty and integrity to improve the health and wellbeing of the local population; reduction of emergency admissions to hospital; transformation of community services including mental health, learning disabilities, dementia and older people services. This is designed to ensure that they are safely and effectively delivered by providing ease of access while maintaining a strong, collaborative focus towards safeguarding people.

Collaboration, when considered alongside such individual, team and organisational developmental milestones (as we have continued to advocate for throughout this chapter) is the primary catalysts for establishing a shared identity; for offering creative practice and innovation: using shared experiences and knowledge to increase team strengths and assist in identifying shared needs: using differing perspectives to identify service gaps more readily: reducing mistrust and professional rivalry and most importantly promoting interprofessional cohesion that proactively promotes reclamation of interdependent functioning for the person (Henneman *et al.*, 1985; Whitehead, 2001).

Conclusions

What is abundantly evident from these variations on collaborative community-based team and organisational perspectives striving to work together across professional boundaries is that goodwill alone will not produce collaboration and the recurring structural impediments that have so often hindered effective opportunities to develop collaborative working. These are all too often related to engrained policy differences; planning and budgetary differences; professional differences and cultural differences that have continued to coexist despite the plethora of current policy drivers, government initiatives and subsequent enactments of legislation (Bamford, 1990; Hudson *et al.*, 1997; Hudson, 2002; Kearney *et al.*, 2003; Quinney, 2006).

Effective collaboration is not merely about fudging the boundaries between the professions, the person with the mental health problems (whose life this is all about after all) or those closest to them, as a consequence of trying to create a generic, one size fits all perspective to mental health and social care practice. Rather, it is about developing people who are confident in their own core skills and are prepared, and willing, to share their expertise and who are fully aware of, and confident in the skills and expertise of their fellow colleagues, to conduct their own practices in a nonhierarchical and collegiate way with members of the team to continuously improve outcomes for people living in their own communities to eventually realise *their* true aspirations and potential, en route to reclaiming their own sense of recovery of interdependent functioning (Hardy, 1999).

References

Bamford, T. (1990) *The Future of Social Work*. Macmillan, Basingstoke.

Barker, P.J. (1990) The philosophy of psychiatric nursing. *Nursing Standard*, 5 (12), 28–33.

Barr, H. (2002) *Interprofessional Education: Yesterday, Today and Tomorrow*. UK Centre for Advancement of Interprofessional Education, University of Westminster.

Barrett, G. & Keeping, C. (2005) The processes required for effective inter professional working. In: *Interprofessional Working in Health and Social Care* (eds G. Barrett, D. Sellman & J. Thomas) Palgrave, Basingstoke.

Braye, S. & Preston-Shoot, M. (2001) *Empowering Practice in Social Care*. Open University Press, Buckingham.

Centre for the Advancement of Interprofessional Education (CAIPE) (1997) *Interprofessional Education: A Fefinition*, CAIPE Bulletin No.13. CAIPE, London.

Clark, C. (2000) *Social Work Ethics: Politics, Principles and Practice*. Macmillan, Basingstoke.

Department of Health (1983) *Mental Health Act*. HMSO, London.

Department of Health (1997) *The Care Programme Approach for People with Mental Illness*. HMSO, London.

Department of Health (1999) *National Service Framework for Mental Health: Modern Standards and Service Models*. The Stationery Office, London.

Department of Health (2000) *No Secrets*, HMSO, London.

Department of Health (2005a) *Mental Capacity Act*. HMSO, London.

Department of Health (2005b) *Ten Essential Shared Capabilities: A Framework for the Whole Mental Health Workforce*. HMSO, London.

Department of Health (2007) *The Mental Health Act 2007*. HMSO, London.

Department of Health (2011) *Health & Social Care Act*. HMSO, London.

Department of Health and Social Security (DoHSS) (1959) *The Mental Health Act 1959*. DHSS, London.

Hardy, J. (ed.) (1999) *Achieving Health and Social Care Improvements through Interprofessional Education. Conference proceedings*. Institute of Health and Community Studies, Bournemouth University.

Henneman, E.A. Lee, J.L. & Cohen, J.I. (1985) Collaboration: a concept analysis. *Journal of Advanced Nursing.* **21**, 103–109.

Hornby, S. & Atkinson, J. (2000) *Collaborative Care: Interprofessional, Interagency and Interpersonal*, 2nd edn. Blackwell Science, Oxford.

Hudson, B. (2002) Interprofessionality in health and social care: the achilles' heel of partnership. *Journal of Interprofessional Care*, **16** (1), 7–17.

Hudson, B., Hardy, B., Henwood, M. & Wistow, G. (1997) *Interagency Collaboration: Final Report*. Nuffield Institute for Health, Leeds.

Kearney, P., Levin, E. & Rosen, G. (2003) *Families that have Alcohol and Mental Health Problems: A Template for Partnership Working*. SCIE, London.

Lord Laming (2003) *The Victoria Climbe Inquiry*. HMSO, Norwich.

Meads, D.G., Chesterton, D., Goosey, D. & Whittington, C. (2003) Practice into theory: learning to facilitate new health and social care partnerships in London. *Learning in Health and Social Care*, **2** (2), 123–136.

Quinney, A. (2006) *Collaborative Social Work*. Learning Matters, Exeter.

Social Care Institute of Excellence (SCIE) (2012) *Think Family*. SCIE, London.

Whitehead, D. (2001) Applying collaborative practice to health promotion. *Nursing Standard.* **15** (20), 33–37.

Williams, P. & Dale, C. (2001) The application of values in working with patients in forensic mental health settings. In: *Forensic Mental Health: Issues in Practice* (eds C. Dale, T. Thompson, & P. Woods). pp. 139–145. BallierreTindall/RCN, Edinburgh.

Section 3

Thriving

Chapter 11

Relationships and Recovery

Stephan D. Kirby

Teesside University, UK

Central to the success or failure of recovery – be it the microfocus of individual treatment activities or the macroprocess of metal health recovery – is the powerful dynamic that is the relationship between the person with mental health problems and the mental health practitioner – the therapeutic bond (Bachelor & Hovarth, 1999). This is the foundation for the effective mutual learning environment within which the person can travel the road of, and towards, recovery with the mental health professional as a companion. Without such a relationship, the person cannot take responsibility and ownership for their mental health problems. This necessitates the need to work as partners in this endeavour. Mental health care practitioners need to remember that health care, especially with people who experience mental health problems is a developmental human activity, through which people (both parties in the venture) learn and grow. Any, and all, relationships in this should be focused upon helping the person with mental health problems and as such are rooted firmly in and focused upon experiences in everyday life.

Mental health practitioners and people with mental health problems are, through working collaboratively in an effective relationship, engaging in a process of mutual influence. A process where any feature or notion of 'us and them' is a false and damaging stance and need eradicating from the outset. A process whose focus is on helping people begin their recovery journey, and we all pursue similar journeys; journeys of discovery.

The responsibility of working in such a collaborative manner is to ensure that we, as mental health practitioner and partners in the therapeutic work, learn from the person's experiences through the facilitation of a dynamic mutual learning environment and work with the person with the mental health problem to (to borrow a term form Narrative Therapy), reauthor their lives, by confronting and healing past distress, through alleviating present distress and thus opening ways to further development (White & Epstein, 1990).

This chapter will discuss the relationship between the person with the mental health problems and the mental health practitioner and the creation of the therapeutic bond (Bachelor & Hovarth, 1999) and how this is actualised as a therapeutic *alliance*. It will then go on to discuss a model of therapeutic alliance in mental health care recovery; a five-phase continuum that utilises the combined essences of recovery and the therapeutic alliance, when working with the person with mental health problems (Kirby, 2001; Kirby & Cross, 2002). This will illustrate how to chart and understand the person's mental health career, as equal partners with and how this is founded on dynamic mutual learning.

This model has also been taken and adapted by the editors to help create their own model of recovery and can be seen in Chapter 14.

Finally, to set the scene, I offer the following:

The therapeutic alliance is the powerful joining of forces which energises and supports the long, difficult and frequently painful work of life changing therapy (Bugental, 1987).

Inherent in every person there is a natural healing impulse, a motivation toward health and wholeness. This motivation can be ignited and strengthened in an environment where an attitude of hope and a belief in each person's potential for growth is pervasive. At the heart of an individual's recovery from mental disorder is the restoration of personal, social, and environmental connections (Barker, 2001:238).

During their training, mental health and social care professionals are immersed in the rhetoric of promoting multiple philosophical and practical models, therapeutic approaches and discourses that promote interprofessional working. Such models and discourses are designed to oppose and challenge the dominance of the medical model and its disease focus to treatment and labelling. However, once in the practice setting, either on student placements or as qualified practitioners, they encounter systems and organisations that reflect (and in doing so, perpetuate) the patriarchal nature of psychiatry and the methods of surveillance and control. As a consequence, practice becomes reduced to methods that reflect oppression and social exclusion (Tee *et al.*, 2012). This paternalistic view infantilises and pathologises people and keeps them in a state of dependency (Barker, 1990). Foucault (1977) succinctly demonstrated how such institutions, designated as caring, are also (or merely) expressions of power, which is exerted over the marginalised groups they are designed to care for by the dominant group, in this case, the Mental Health Practitioner. Despite progress in service development, design, focus and delivery, this is still relevant and prevalent in the twenty-first century, in fact possibly more so. This is due to the fact that the once visible power of the large mental hospitals of recent years (despite the safety and security offered to the incumbent person with mental health problems by the buildings and organisational structures) has been replaced by control and power enacted through policy and enforced by bureaucracy to a mental health service that is characterised by its community focus to care delivery that is fragmented, compartmentalised and fundamentally risk averse.

It is not surprising therefore that concerns are consistently being raised from people with mental health problems and the associated user groups that mental health professionals are not being taught the correct and necessary skills and are becoming less, rather than more, conversant with the day-to-day practical concerns of people with mental health problems. They continue to claim that no-one is listening to them (Kirby & Cross, 2002). Indeed, perceptions of in-patient mental health care suggests that mental health practitioners are spending less time relating to their charges and more time in office-related administration. Regardless of the type of setting or service where mental health care is taking place, it is essential that practitioners are continually sensitive to the barriers that constrain and obstruct a free two-way communication and discourse. Having an awareness of, and applying actions that counter, the differences between *having* power (even beneficial power) over another and *sharing* power with a treatment partner are essential. In a service where an asylum mentality still prevails, the worse aspect of power that mental health professionals hold over people with mental health problems is the power of denial (Campbell, 1998).

Many practitioners are employed in traditional settings working within traditional organisational frameworks and treatment models and approaches to engagement and recovery; in other words, within settings where psychiatry (and all that entails) is the organisation. This culture where patriarchal psychiatry is still dominant; where the medical model is still very evident is in opposition to, rather than the dominant option of, an ethos of mental health professionals working in partnership towards a mutually determined goal by mutually determined methods and within appropriate mutually determined timescales (Trenoweth *et al.*, 2011). People with mental health problems continue to state that they wish, indeed *need*, to be informed, supported and encouraged to participate and collaborate in their own care. There is a clear relationship between the extent to which people feel able to discuss their concerns and care with mental health care professionals and their subsequent agreement with treatment and care regimes.

The competencies for Mental Health Nursing (NMC, 2010) consistently and repeatedly state that the therapeutic use of self is central to a nursing professional's, and therefore *all* mental health practitioners, ability to promote mental health wellbeing with their charges. What the therapeutic use of self suggests that we need to use 'who' we are as a healing influence in our relationships with people with mental health problems (Tee *et al.*, 2012). Therefore to demonstrate that they are effective and competent in their practice, mental health practitioners of all disciplines need to acquire and promote an emancipatory stance. Individual practitioners need to critically examine their values; adopt a more sceptical position and challenge the dominant discourse, therefore challenging its validity; examine their workplace culture and contribute to a process of cultural change (Tee *et al.*, 2012). This changed culture would support and reflect people's desire to be informed, supported and encouraged to participate and therefore collaborate in their own care (Trenoweth *et al.*, 2011). In this sense, it is (or should be) obvious that collaboration is more than 'mere' good practice (NICE, 2009). It is the stance by which any helping relationship is influenced by the person's view of how relevant the intervention is to them and how effective it is likely to be (Trenoweth *et al.*, 2011) as they become more involved in their own care.

In (relatively) recent years, mental health practitioners have started to come out from the shadow of the paternalistic medical model and medically dominant establishment where care is often viewed as something we do *to* people rather than *with* people (Barker, 1990). This approach to mental health care arose from a desire to control the 'mentally ill' person and thus remain litigation averse. There is now a greater focus on the person with mental health problems as an individual not as a collection of complex pathologies. Contemporary mental health care needs to continue to evolve in order to remain responsive to the needs of not only a changing society but also the rapidly changing care arena. This responsiveness is directly mirrored within, and a mirror image of, society's (frequently negative) views towards mental health; the people with mental health problems as well as the health care professionals. This is regularly fuelled by media feeding frenzies that occur during and following high profile inquiries.

Historically, mental health practitioners were discouraged by their qualified, supposedly more experienced, superiors from forming what they termed 'personal', 'special' or 'individual' relationships with people with mental health problems. We were told that we did not need to, nor should we, become 'too involved' with *them*. We are now aware that the interpersonal relationship represents the proper focus of practice; especially mental health, and a practitioner's therapeutic strength lies in their ability to enhance a person's restoration of rational, life enhancing growth: in other words, empowerment (Kirby & Cross, 2002).

Mental health practice raises dilemmas that the professional must wrestle with on a daily basis, none more problematic than having and maintaining the ethical principle of respect for people (Swinton & Boyd, 2000). This is fundamental to mental health care as professionals should retain respect for people, irrespective of their capacities, capabilities, social status, any offending profile, behaviour or values. This places all human being as equals; places them on an equal level and gives them equivalent rights and responsibilities based on the understanding that as 'persons' they have a worth (Kirby & Cross, 2002). This principle calls on professionals to ensure that people with mental health problems are treated as people with relational, spiritual and material needs (Swinton & Boyd, 2000). Mental health professionals care for vulnerable people who may be thought disordered; may have relationship difficulties or may be emotionally fragile and thus multiprofessional, multidisciplinary, mental health care remains a fundamentally relational enterprise. Having the ability to be a companion with a sense of fairness and humanity is essential, as these qualities are particularly effective in helping people find a sense of affinity with professionals. It is based on the principle of people relating to other people and it is through that relationship that forms of healing and/or relief from psychological or physical disorder are arrived at (Swinton & Boyd, 2000). This is an integral part of the therapeutic and person-centred process. Such provision is a dynamic process; a mutual and dynamic learning process by which all involved can, and will, benefit.

We need to encourage and assist people with mental health problems to take a greater responsibility for their mental health problems and the way they affect and impact upon their lives and not to negate this responsibility by handing it to the mental health professionals. We (as professionals) encourage this in a misguided notion of feeling wanted and needed by people with mental health problems. We *are* needed and wanted but not to tell them what to do and/or what not to do, nor to prescribe their care for them; rather we are needed by them as partners to work together, in an alliance, to reach a mutually agreed resolution of the problem areas. How can we profess to know 'what to do' *for* people with mental health problems when we are not affected and nor need assistance in seeking resolution. Irrespective of discipline, professionals have a responsibility for maintaining the safety of people with mental health problems and adapting the physical and organisational care environment to enhance the promotion of person-centred health (mental and physical).

While having a desire to exercise more personal control and have a greater involvement in the decision making process regarding whether, or not, they receive treatment and its nature, most people who have mental health problems would not want to exercise power over individual mental health professionals (Barnes & Bowl, 2001); unfortunately, the same cannot be said of the reverse situation. People with mental health problems are no longer content to be the mere recipients of helpful yet planned interventions they wish to be listened to and understood as well as to be involved in the planning of the care and the clinical decision-making process. They do not want to be able to learn how to just manage better; they want to feel better too.

The collaborative nature of mental health expects, and demands, care provision where the alliances between people with mental health problems and professionals are the cornerstones of the treatment process. This not only promotes a culture of empowerment where the person takes more responsibility for their lives and actions but also supports and facilitates greater engagement with their condition (Watson & Kirby, 2000). Engagement within the collaborative therapeutic alliance can be threatening to all parties concerned. People in mental health services have often had little active involvement in their own care. For some, this will be a welcome and refreshing change but for others the increased responsibility can be quite daunting and unwelcome. Many may feel quite hopeless about the prospect of change whilst others will be weighed down by low motivation. An emphasis on individual empowerment must remain one of the fundamental principles of care as it lies at the heart of the caring process (Kirby & Cross, 2002). Therefore, the therapeutic alliance is an essential and potentially powerful vehicle within which personal responsibility is promoted and monitored.

The therapeutic alliance

The therapeutic alliance is seen as 'the glue' that binds the person with the mental health problem and the practitioner together (Bachelor & Hovarth, 1999) and permits them to work together in a realistic, collaborative relationship that is based on mutual respect, liking and trust as well as an equal commitment to the activities of treatment. Three components have been proposed (Bordin, 1979) as being essential to an effective therapeutic alliance: 'interpersonal bonds', 'agreement on the goals of treatment' and 'collaboration on therapeutic tasks'. Part of the person's essential personal growth process involves an increased awareness and acceptance of their own problems, so that problem solving can occur (Bordin, 1979). Therefore, the therapeutic alliance is just one element of an integrated psychological approach to mental health care. It is obvious that caring for people with mental health problems cannot occur in the absence of a therapeutic alliance.

Effective relationships within the therapeutic alliance are distinguished by their dynamic mutual learning process. This fundamental concept is utilised by both parties; the person with the mental health problem helps the practitioner to understand (in their own words) how they conceptualise, rationalise, explain and cope with their mental health problems (e.g., hearing voices, depression and anger/aggression problems) and consequently the practitioner learns from these expressions of the person's experiences – both positive and negative. This allows them to enter into modes of treatment that are both meaningful and contextual and that will continue to promote deeper learning through their individuality and focus (Kirby & Cross, 2002).

The commonest form of disempowerment involves the failure to afford a proper hearing to the person with mental health problem's story of the experiences of their problems of living (Barker, 2001). By working collaboratively in a therapeutic alliance, it is possible for people with mental health problems (and their carers) and mental health care professionals to develop an alternative, theoretically based approach to care delivery. This is grounded in the sharing of life experiences through narrative approaches ('to know madness we have to get inside the experience'); the sharing of decision-making and problem-solving techniques; and the construction and sharing of a mutual language and discourse that supports (mutual) empowerment. The expertise of the person with the mental health problem as direct consumers has only been partially exploited, and their obvious expertise in 'madness' has barely been explored. Respect for the insights of 'mad persons' would not only be useful and essential, it would also be courteous to our therapeutic partners (Campbell, 1998).

So at the heart of adopting, and engaging in, a therapeutic alliance is the understanding that the only way mental health professionals can be of real benefit to the person with mental health problems is to learn from their experiences and facilitate a dynamic learning process whereby the professionals learn what to do *for* the person, *from* the person (Barker, 1995). This learning process is one of the most crucial elements in building any form of social relationship with anyone. We must develop our ability, and willingness, to understand life as it is from the other person's stance; from their perspective. Although it is never possible to know what life is *exactly* like for someone else, a willingness to explore the way the person with mental health problems sees their situation is essential.

The mental health professional must understand the diverse range of ways in which people function, behave and interact when *they are* mentally disordered. A key aspect of developing a therapeutic alliance is engendering a trusting capacity. One of the key beliefs of this alliance is that 'people are not the problem – the problem is the problem' (White & Epstein, 1990; Barker, 1995) and if professionals do anything of worth with their interactions it has to be to offer hope. They hold out a 'hopeline' to people who are often devoid of hope (Barker, 1990). Hope is an 'anticipation of a continued good state, an improved state of release from a perceived entrapment'. Maintaining hope is a challenge of the person with mental health problems, and the therapeutic alliance is seen to be the most powerful 'hope instilling' strategy available when working with damaged and the vulnerable people as so many of us do (Repper & Perkins, 2003).

The professional's attitude towards both the person with mental health problems and the successful formation of the alliance is as important as the therapeutic techniques employed. Nothing should take precedence over the best interests of the person with mental health problems, and the professional must be convinced of and continually strive to ensure the effectiveness of what they are doing within the alliance. This can only be provided through the use of an empirically sound and research-based approach to care within the therapeutic alliance.

Prior to entering into such a therapeutic alliance, the metal health professional must ask themselves,

'...can I permit myself to enter into the private world(s) of this person, explore their feelings without judging them, and in some significant and honest way, respond in a manner that lets them know that I have listened and I want to provide whatever assistance or comfort that I can?';

'...can I see this person as being unique in his/her reaction to mental health problems?';

'...can I see what is different, and the same, about this person so that any insight or assistance I may give is the most useful to this person?' (Safran *et al.*, 1990).

It is within such an alliance that the person with mental health problems is being given the opportunity to develop a sense of control where they are involved as an active participant. They have a positive relationship with the mental health professional (which includes and is characterised by warmth, friendship, empathy, respect and concern) and be certain of receiving timely and relevant information and feedback, and this can be done through being involved in the discussion and negotiation of mutual expectations and the clarification of rights and responsibilities of both parties (Speedy, 1999).

Central to the therapeutic alliance approach is the use of discourse and reflexivity as therapeutic mediums (Rorty, 1979). While discourse is a 'conversation with others' and a 'social process', reflexivity is the 'capacity of any system to turn back upon itself, to make its own object by referring to itself' (Ruby, 1982). By being reflexive, we make ourselves the object of our own observations, and the person with mental health problems is able to 'step aside' from the discourse/conversation they were initially engaged in and view it from another perspective (Lax, 1992). To provide an effective, meaningful and dynamic therapeutic alliance, the mental health professional needs to ensure the continued use of reflection throughout the therapeutic process. Both their own reflections as well as encouraging the other person to engage in a reflective process. Therefore, having a robust reflexive and narrative foundation is an important aspect of the integrated partnership approach for the therapeutic alliance.

The therapeutic alliance needs to be carried out in the context of interprofessional working and the multidisciplinary team. Therefore, training in the necessary narrative focused intervention strategies is imperative. As the proposed therapeutic alliance will be very challenging, mental health professionals must ensure that high quality and appropriate clinical and academic supervision is available and utilised throughout practical application of any intervention strategies.

The role of the mental health professional within the therapeutic alliance must be one of encouragement, providing incentive, clarification and offering rationales for what is expected from the person with mental health problems. That said, there is no magic in developing a therapeutic alliance. It does, however, require hard work, courage and insight for both parties involved. Both individuals in a therapeutic alliance desire to be accepted, liked and respected *and* both individuals want to accept, like and respect the other. An effective therapeutic alliance is only possible when the professional is seen as competent, trustworthy and caring.

Elements of the user group movement (e.g., Survivors Speak Out; UK Advocacy Network [UKAN]) over the years have continued to campaign for a greater emphasis to be giving to empowerment in mental health care. The objectives of such groups include promoting personal empowerment through increased value being given to the experiences and knowledge's of people with mental health problems as well as by strengthening the social networks for people with mental health problems. They claim they seek empowerment within the mental health system by challenging professional control and demonstrating alternative models of support for people experiencing mental distress (Barnes & Bowl, 2001). They desire a presence at national level in order to exert more political influence on mental health policy makers.

Power within the mental health arena comes from two forces, the person with the mental health problem and the authority; the organisationally imposed power placed on the mental health professional. These invariably meet head on and lock horns in immediate confrontation. Such confrontation is based on the premise that one set of ideals, beliefs and behaviours come into conflict with, and against, another. While one set of ideals (rules) set out to control, through compliancy and conformity, and the application and demonstration of power, the other seeks to survive this, through maintaining as much autonomy and personal freedom as is possible (no matter how little that may be). The ideals and belief systems coming into conflict are the rules binding their behaviours, the behaviours of authority and domination and the behaviours of resistance and survival (Kirby, 2010).

Empowerment should be understood as a process in which people develop the 'power' to take decisions; take actions; make choices and/or work with others where they have so far been unable to do so (Barnes & Bowl, 2001). This is built on the essential premise of not involving or utilising coercive power to make people do things. It is one of the central practical concerns for all practitioners when endeavouring to deliver effective alliance-based mental health care. We have a unique capacity to influence and assist people with mental health problems in living through, and living with, their distress on a daily basis. The extent to which professionals are prepared to share power is critical both practically and morally. It is clear that persons with mental health problems and mental health practitioners are now talking and listening together more. What is questionable however is both the quality of the interactions and the boundaries of the topics being debated. Are we functioning at a therapeutic and meaningful level or merely providing an outlet for social discourse? (Rorty, 1979). Interpersonal relations are the proper focus of mental health care and therapeutic strength lies the professionals ability to enhance a person's empowerment (Kirby, 2001), though we need to continually remind ourselves that mental health professionals cannot empower people with mental health problems rather only people with mental health problems can empower people with mental health problems (Barker, 1995).

A model of therapeutic alliance in mental health recovery

Therapeutic alliance; working alliance or helping alliance have been used, sometimes interchangeably, to describe the relationship that must exist between a mental health professional and a person with mental health problems within which positive therapeutic change takes place (Foreman & Marmar, 1985). The therapeutic alliance is the concept and framework within which the mental health professional and the person with mental health problems work together in a realistic, collaborative relationship. This is based on mutual respect, liking, trust and commitment to the work of treatment (Foreman & Marmar, 1985). This alliance is the product of the combined and unified determination brought by the person and professionals and their ability to work together on aspects of the person's relationships with others and the multiple realities caused by an 'illness' symptomatology. Part of the person's growth process involves an increased awareness and acceptance of their own problems, so that problem solving can occur. Successful therapy cannot take place without such an alliance, which is equivalent to a working relationship in any team effort outside the therapeutic setting (Kirby & Cross, 2002). Partnership negotiation and shared decision making are necessary to underpin the relationship within the alliance. It must be made clear that, as such, shared decision making diverges quite markedly from compliance. Whereas compliance (to decisions made, and within, treatment approaches) is used to increase a person's conformity, shared decision making assumes that two experts (the person with the mental health problem and the mental health practitioner) must share their expertise, their respective information and determine collaboratively the optimal treatment (Deegan & Drake, 2006). Thus, there is a continually growing move beyond paternalistic compliance (rooted as it is within the medical model) to the therapeutic alliance (Deegan & Drake, 2006). The movement that is taking place of moving from compliance and towards shared decision making entails a process of collaboration which will result in arriving at a mutually acceptable plan for moving the treatment agenda forward. The mental health practitioner's role is not to ensure compliance but rather to help the person with the mental health problem to learn and through the process of learning to manage how their experiences of mental health problems affect their life. It becomes obvious therefore that within a shared decision-making approach the language and mindset of medical authority, compliance with therapy and coercive treatments disappears and concepts like education, individual experience, informed choice, collaborative experts and self management of mental health problems take over.

A model of practice utilising the therapeutic alliance is thus proposed, and this initiates and develops a mutual learning dynamic which makes it possible for the knowledge(s), experience(s) and insights of both people with mental health problems and mental health professional to be drawn on when mutually developing problem solving strategies (Kirby, 2001; Kirby & Cross, 2002). Such a model will not only produce better therapeutic outcomes for the person but will also provide learning opportunities for the professionals to further develop practice (Marsh & Fisher, 1992). Both the person with mental health problems and mental health professional can benefit as a result (Barnes & Bowl, 2001). One of the advantageous effects of this new inclusive and empowering clinical situation is that people with mental health problems are coming to realise that they have a voice and viewpoint and a legitimate entitlement to be heard.

The terms 'therapeutic alliance' and 'therapeutic relationship' convey similar meanings; however, the alliance, particularly within the context of this particular model, also includes a mutual and shared (by both person with mental health problems and mental health professional) understanding of the meanings given by the person of their behaviour in any given situation. The therapeutic alliance is also distinguished by the pendulous nature of the decision making and therapeutic and professional power (Kirby, 2001; Kirby & Cross, 2002). This is evidenced by the way the power agenda and ownership and usage of power within the alliance swings from one individual to the other and is constantly changing as the nature and focus of the therapy changes. For there are always times and situations where shared decision making is not always fully applicable (Deegan & Drake, 2006), for example, in times of mental health crisis and in such situations the decision making and therapeutic power will lie with the professional but always with the best interests of the person with the mental health problem at the forefront. This will continue until the person is more able to regain and retake their part in the shared decision making of the therapeutic alliance. In the context of such a therapeutic alliance, one that is characterised by the absence of threat and by the presence of mutual encouragement and comfort, people with mental health problems do eventually feel sufficiently safe and courageous to tackle hitherto neglected aspects of their experience and life (Kirby, 2001).

This particular model of therapeutic alliance for mental health care is depicted as and can be understood and actioned by the implementation of, a continuum with identifiable stages. These commence at the person with mental health problems first contact with the service and the practitioner(s) (*Entry into the Mental Health System*), and progress towards an ultimate state of improved self management, and increased levels of autonomy and engagement, which are appropriate to their environment and level of functioning, towards and through recovery (*Return to Social World*). In order to achieve progression along this continuum, the following phases are engaged with throughout the recovery journey (Kirby, 2001; Kirby & Cross, 2002).

Survival – maintaining existence and surviving the risk associated with critical times of acute mental distress;

Reconstruction – a time of personal change, where the person finds new ways to live and cope more effectively with their mental health problems through the development of new interpersonal skills and problem solving approaches;

Growth – a time of increasing self knowledge, greater social awareness and understanding relating to the person's mental health problems;

Recovery – developing an increasing level of functioning to allow the person to take more involvement and responsibility for their own mental health care;

Reintegration – this is the final phase, when the person is able to demonstrate their full potential relating to self management skills and optimum levels and methods of empowerment to safeguard their mental health and rejoin their social world. (This is described in further detail in the aforementioned Kirby, 2001; Kirby & Cross, 2002)

It is worth pointing out briefly that the sequence of the original phases in this model of therapeutic alliance has changed slightly since the original 2001 and 2002 publications. This reflects a process that is more proactive in its approach to, and engagement with, the recovery process; one where the focus is firmly on personal growth and development, interprofessional working and recovery.

The issue of interpersonal boundaries is fundamental to the success of the therapeutic process for the protection of both the practitioner and the person and also to aid therapeutic progress. At the outset, the relationship between the person with mental health problems and the mental health professionals is relatively neutral with clear boundaries dictated by professional standards, power ownership and cultural expectation. Boundaries within professional practice are used to define mutual acceptable conduct and limits of practice (Kirby, 2001). Within such a therapeutic alliance, the mental health practitioner needs to be clear about the boundaries of the relationship, the power issues, rules of confidentiality and the duty of care. The extent to which practitioners are prepared to exercise power over people with mental health problems or to share it with them is critical in both a practical and a moral sense (Kirby, 2001). Mental health practitioners need to examine how their practice maintains the powerlessness of people with mental health problems, as this will inevitably lead to the long-term damaging of individuals (Kirby, 2001).

Within this strategic approach to care which adopts and utilises the therapeutic alliance, is the application of psychoeducational interventions developed within a framework of integrated psychological approaches for the treatment of mental health problems (Cross & Kirby, 2002).

Psycho-educational interventions combine educational and therapeutic objectives and offer material about the mental health problem and therapeutic strategies, which are designed to reduce the person's possibility of relapse (Solomon, 1996). Stress and burden are reduced by the application of interventions that are focused upon improving a person's quality of life. Second, there is, as importantly, a need to help relatives and friends cope with difficult situations and support the person with mental health problems in their care programmes.

Psychoeducation can be seen as very much part of partnership working within the therapeutic alliance. It addresses issues of people with mental health problems and on the impact their mental health problems have on interpersonal behaviours and relationships (Cross & Kirby, 2002). It also provides a model that empowers (Hayes & Gnatt, 1992). It appears that psychoeducation provides a sense of dignity and self-esteem as practitioners trust people with mental health problems with information and place the tools for self-care in their hands (Cross & Kirby, 2002). It requires people to engage with, and participate in, their treatment, rather than being merely passive recipients or even adversaries. The knowledge and skills learned through psychoeducation clarifies for people how they understand the extent(s) of their mental health problems. This empowers them to become who they are; to be more than a 'schizophrenic', rather to be a person with problems, who has the same life tasks ahead of them as does everyone else (Cross & Kirby, 2002). Psychoeducation involves the practitioner working collaboratively with the person and their families and carers. Such interventions are characteristically open and honest within the confines of a professional relationship underpinned by a therapeutic alliance. The person with mental health problem's abilities to participate in psychoeducational interventions serve to set the guide, the pace of the process. If individuals are not able to participate in the psychoeducational activities nor willing to make decisions about their lives, it will be very difficult to proceed. When using psychoeducational techniques they should be inherently motivating, so that the person finds them interesting and this encourages people to join in because they see the rationale behind it; that being personal growth and development (Cross & Kirby, 2002).

Conclusions

In order to develop our approaches to mental health care, we need to acknowledge the need for change and embrace change activities. In doing so, and to remain effective, we need to develop 'new' skills and learn 'new' therapeutic models. The model (continuum) of therapeutic alliances discussed briefly here promotes the premise that mental health care is effective when the person (person with mental health problems or mental health professional) begins to experience growth and development through developing, and engaging in, a dynamic, mutual learning process. This approach allows, indeed encourages, the mental health professional to develop safe boundaries to their practice while maintaining the freedom to develop ethical and inclusive, effective and knowledgeable, flexible and collaborative interventions that will, ultimately, become the future focus of their practice (Cross & Kirby, 2002).

It is hoped that people with mental health problems will benefit from this approach as a result of a more integrated, encompassing and effective care delivery package. At the centre of this is respect for the person's individuality and that the therapeutic alliance is intensified through the practitioner's adoption and utilisation of alternative knowledge bases. The mental health professional will have greater understanding of, and engage more effectively with, the experience(s) of their mental health problems, which should result in increased motivation and job satisfaction for the professional and greater and more beneficial therapeutic outcomes for the person with mental health problems.

Such understandings of the nature of the 'problem creating experience' are prerequisite for successful self-management and coping. Therefore, it is critical that mental health practitioners develop a greater understanding of alternative knowledge bases that explore representations of self and other, the individual and the social and cultural environment in which they all exist (Kirby, 2001; Cross & Kirby, 2002; Kirby & Cross, 2002). The future of collaboratively focused, recovery-based, mental health care is through the effective use of therapeutic alliances and a more interpersonal focus to our care strategies. We must embrace the benefits that can be gained from utilising alternative knowledge bases; those alternative to the dominant and all pervasive medical model.

Finally, Fee (2000) considers that this is time to reconnect the pathological to the rapidly shifting, material, cultural and psychosocial realms of life and likewise to alter our theoretical and methodological frameworks to better understand such connections.

References

Bachelor, A. & Hovarth, A. (1999) The therapeutic relationship. In: *The Heart and Soul of Change: What Works in Therapy* (eds M.A. Hubble, B.L. Duncan & S.D. Miller), pp. 133–178. American Psychological Association, Washington, DC.

Barker, P.J. (1990) The philosophy of psychiatric nursing. *Nursing Standard*, **5** (12), 28–33.

Barker, P.J. (1995) *Healing Lives, Mending Minds: Professorial Inaugural Lecture.* University of Newcastle, Newcastle.

Barker, P.J. (2001) The Tidal Model: developing an empowering, person centred approach to recovery within psychiatric and mental health nursing. *Journal of Psychiatric and Mental Health Nursing,* **8,** 233–240.

Barnes, M. & Bowl, R. (2001) *Taking Over the Asylum: Empowerment and Mental Health.* Palgrave, Basingstoke.

Bordin, E.S. (1979) The generalisability of the psychoanalytic concept of the working alliance. *Psychotherapy: Theory, Research and Practice,* **16,** 252–260.

Bugental, J. (1987) *The Art of the Psychotherapist.* Norton, New York.

Campbell P. (1998) Listening to clients. In: *Psychiatric Nursing: Ethical Strife* (eds P.J. Barker & B. Davison), pp. 237–248. Arnold, London.

Cross, D.J. & Kirby, S.D. (2002) Using psychoeducational interventions within an integrated psychological approach to forensic mental health and social care. In: *Therapeutic Interventions for Forensic Mental Health Nurses* (eds A.M. Kettles, P. Woods & M. Collins), pp. 72–91. Jessica Kingsley Publishers, London.

Deegan, P.E. & Drake, R.E. (2006) Shared decision making and medication management in the recovery process. *Psychiatric Services,* **57** (11), 1636–1639.

Fee, D. (ed.) (2000) *Pathology and the Postmodern: Mental Illness as Discourse and Experience.* Sage, London.

Foreman S.A. & Marmar, C.R. (1985) Therapist action that addresses initially poor therapeutic alliances in psychotherapy. *American Journal of Psychotherapy,* **142,** 922–926.

Foucault, M. (1977) *Discipline and Punish: The Birth of the Prison.* Penguin, London.

Hayes, R. & Gnatt, A. (1992) Patient psychoeducation: The therapeutic use of knowledge for the mentally ill. *Social Work in Health Care,* **17** (1), 53–67.

Kirby, S.D. (2001) The development of a conceptual framework of therapeutic alliance in psychiatric (nursing) care delivery. In: *Forensic Mental Health: Working with the Mentally Ill Offender* (eds G. Landsberg & A. Smiley). pp. 25:1–25:8. Civic Research Institute, Kingston.

Kirby, S.D. (2010) *What is the Meaning of Segregation for Prisoners: Creating a Space for Survival by Reframing Contextual Power* Unpublished PhD Thesis, Teesside University, Middlesbrough.

Kirby, S.D. & Cross, D.J. (2002) Socially constructed narrative intervention: a foundation for therapeutic alliances. In: *Therapeutic Interventions for Forensic Mental Health Nurses* (eds A.M. Kettles, P. Woods & M. Collins). pp. 187–205. Jessica Kingsley Publishers, London.

Lax, W.D. (1992) Postmodern thinking in a clinical practice. In: *Therapy as Social Construction* (eds S. McNamee & K.J. Gergen). pp. 69–85. Sage, London.

Marsh, P. & Fisher, M. (1992) *Good Intentions: Developing Partnership in Social Services.* Joseph Rowntree Foundation, York.

National Institute for Clinical Excellence (NICE) (2009) *Medicines Adherence.* NICE, London.

Nursing and Midwifery Council (NMC) (2010) *Standards for Pre-registration Nursing Education.* NMC, London.

Repper, J. & Perkins, R. (2003) *Social Inclusion and Recovery: A Model for Mental Health Practice.* Elsevier Health Sciences, Edinburgh.

Rorty, R. (1979) *Philosophy and the Mirror of Nature.* Princeton University Press, Princeton.

Ruby, J. (1982) *A Crack in the Mirror*. University of Pennsylvania Press, Philadelphia.

Safran, J.D., McMain, S. & Crocker, P. (1990) Therapeutic alliance rupture as a therapy event for empirical investigation. *Psychotherapy*, **27**, 155–165.

Solomon, P. (1996) Moving from psychoeducation to family education for families of adults with serious mental illness. *Psychiatric Services*, **47**, 1364–1370.

Speedy, S. (1999) The therapeutic alliance. In: *Advanced Practice in Mental Health Nursing* (eds M. Clinton & S. Nelson). Blackwell Science, Oxford.

Swinton, J. & Boyd, J. (2000) Autonomy and personhood: the forensic nurse as a moral agent. In: *Forensic Nursing and Multidisciplinary Care of the Mentally Disordered Offender*. (eds D. Robinson, & A.M. Kettles). pp. 128–141. Jessica Kingsley Publishers, London.

Tee, S., Brown, J. & Carpenter, D. (2012) *Handbook of Mental Health Nursing*. Hodder Arnold, London.

Trenoweth, S., Docherty, T., Franks, J. & Pearce, R. (2011) *Nursing and Mental Health Care: An Introduction for All Fields of Practice*. Learning Matters, Exeter.

Watson, C. & Kirby, S.D. (2000) A two nation perspective on issues of practice and provision for professionals caring for mentally disordered offenders. In: *Forensic Nursing and Multidisciplinary Care of the Mentally Disordered Offender*. (eds D. Robinson & A.M. Kettles). pp. 51–62. Jessica Kingsley Publishers, London.

White, M. & Epston, D. (1990) *Narrative Means to Therapeutic Ends*. Norton, New York.

Chapter 12

Holistic Care Planning for Recovery

Devon Marston[1] and Jenny Weinstein[2]

[1]Channel One Band, UK
[2]Kingston University, UK

Person-centred care planning must involve users and their families, or community carers, in all aspects of care planning; at every stage, care planning must address all aspects of a person's life, not simply their medical condition. In order to comply with the current best practice, the care planning should be underpinned by a Recovery approach (NIMHE, 2005; CSIP, RCP & SCIE, 2007) rather than a traditional medical or social care model.

To demonstrate how some of these principles can be translated into practice and to provide live examples, the authors will be drawing on their own experience of working closely with mental health service users, both in hospital and in the community. Devon Marston, the Wounded Healer, was the founder member of a user-led mental health arts and music organisation called Sound Minds (see www.soundminds.co.uk), and Jenny Weinstein previously worked in partnership with service users in mental health (see Weinstein, 2010) and now campaigns with service users, carers, families and friends, for better services.

The recovery approach

The Recovery approach has fundamentally changed our thinking about mental health and mental illness. It requires professionals to stop seeing service users as ill people who must be looked after and supervised to recognising them as individuals with strengths, hopes and aspirations. It is these strengths, hopes and aspirations that should underpin and inform care planning, which should be user-led. The family or other informal carer should also be involved (Worthington & Rooney, 2010) unless the service user specifically requests that this should not happen. Whether or not the service user

Care Planning in Mental Health: Promoting Recovery, Second Edition.
Edited by Angela Hall, Michael Wren and Stephan D. Kirby.
© 2013 John Wiley & Sons, Ltd. Published 2013 by John Wiley & Sons, Ltd.

wishes their carer or family to be involved, carers and family members have their own needs and entitlements, which should be considered and addressed by mental health professionals.

Key principles underpinning the Recovery approach are set out by the Sainsbury Centre for Mental Health (Shepherd *et al.*, 2008):

- Hope is central to recovery;
- Self-management is encouraged and facilitated;
- The helping relationship between clinicians and patients moves away from being expert/patient to being 'coaches' or 'partners' on a journey of discovery;
- People do not recover in isolation. Recovery is closely associated with social inclusion and being able to take on meaningful and satisfying social roles within local communities rather than in segregated services;
- Recovery is about discovering, or rediscovering, a sense of personal identity, separate from illness or disability.

(Shepherd *et al.*, 2008:1)

Holistic person-centred care planning

In the views of the authors, a user and carer involvement strategy is essential to the implementation of person-centred care planning. According to Simpson and House (2003), 'stakeholder involvement, is an approach in which participants work within the mental health services undertaking a range of roles in addition to participating in planning, developing and monitoring mental health services. Service providers should play an active part in involving users and carers as genuine partners in services' (p. 1266). The following example shows how one Trust involved stakeholders to address the issue of implementing holistic person-centred care planning.

In 2010, a Care Quality Commission (CQC) inspection of a large psychiatric hospital found that care planning was still undertaken mainly on a medical model with insufficient involvement of service users and carers. A workshop was held for service users and other stakeholders to address and resolve the issues. Users said the following about their experiences:

- 'I don't feel I have any choice – I feel like a fly being caught in a spider's web and I can't get out';
- 'You are put in a subservient position and what *they* think is imposed on you';
- 'No-one wants to know what our aspirations are or asks what would be useful to us'.

Barriers to person-centred care planning

Workshop participants were asked to identify the barriers that prevented holistic, person-centred care planning, and the following issues were raised:

- Process that is top down not bottom up;
- Carers are not involved or informed;
- No choices or options given on treatment or medication;
- Current way process is set up, making it just a tick-box exercise;
- Staff attitudes still focus on a diagnosis and treatment – not on the whole person;
- Cultural and social conditioning about mental illness persists;
- Management are not committed enough to make sure it happens – no senior person owns responsibility;
- Staff are not trained in person-centred or recovery approaches. They regard care planning simply as 'paperwork';
- The requirements and protocols make it difficult to have a human-to-human conversation because of the pro forma rules;
- The complexities involved in mental ill health are hard to capture;
- The risk averse/obsessed culture overrides everything;
- The electronic recording system uses a medical model.

What would good care planning look like?

Participants were asked how they would recognise good quality care planning, and the following proposals were made:

- It needs to be a living document added to each day, recognising that people or their situation change each day;
- It should begin with the person's view about how they are and their recovery goals and aspirations;
- Advance directives and care plans made in the community should be transferred when a person becomes ill and is admitted and then go back out with them to the community;
- The plan should involve carers, family, friends or anyone important to the user;
- New Care Planning documentation would enable service user access through a secure portal so that they can add to or change their care plan – like a blog.

How can change be achieved?

Participants were asked what they thought needed to happen for real change to be achieved, and the following suggestions were made:

- Staff attitudes would change if training for mental health staff, including doctors, was provided by service users;
- There should be a champion in the Trust who would recruit service users and arrange for them to be trained as trainers;

A holistic response at admission to hospital

The 'Acute Care Declaration' was drawn up by the National Mental Health Development Unit (Stoddart, 2009) to bring in-patient care up to agreed standards.

People who are admitted to hospital are usually quite ill and need skilled medical help, but it is important to remember that, although unwell and even incoherent, people will still be aware of how they are being dealt with and spoken to and this will affect their response to professionals.

When you go into psychiatric hospital for the first time, or any time for that matter, it is still a very frightening experience. A research study undertaken by Abbott *et al.* (2009) indicates that medical and nursing students are often anxious about communicating with patients with mental health problems, even when they have received general communication skills training, but that respect can be shown for patients as autonomous beings. In the author's experience, in many psychiatric hospitals, staff rarely sit down and talk to you in an informal and friendly way on the ward. They give out medicine, they call you for meals, they do 'ward rounds', but they do not take an interest in you as a human being. They may even be on a duty to observe you, but they do not engage. Some staff use the opportunity to sit and read a newspaper or magazine. Holistic care planning should be a starting point for establishing a meaningful and respectful relationship with the patient (Case Example 12.1).

Case Example 12.1

At night I could not sleep despite the medication I had been given. By that time, I had realised that I was in hospital but the chaotic environment was confusing. I could hear people screaming and arguing constantly, staff and patients alike, as if no one was in control. It felt strange because though my head was a bit wobbly, I could remember that hospitals usually feel like places of safety. Besides on the following day, I still had not been told what I was doing there.

(Raptopolous, 2010:75)

Being picked up by the police and put in the back of a police van and taken to hospital on a (section) 136 order is an especially frightening experience. You may not have the clothes or personal effects you need; your family may not know what is happening and even you yourself do not know what is happening. Following any hospital admission, people need reassurance and to have an explanation about what is happening to them. This should include help to understand:

- where you are;
- why you are there;
- what will happen next;
- what your rights are.

Handing someone an explanatory leaflet or, worse still, pointing to something on a notice board is not adequate. Someone needs to sit patiently, listen to questions and concerns and explain to both the service user and a family member or friend who cares for them.

Once you are well enough, someone needs to sit down with you and find out about you as a person: where you live, who you are living with, who are your family members, whether you have dependent children, whether anyone is dependent on you for support, you may be worrying about them. Are you part of a faith community? What do you like to do? – play/watch sport, music, computer, reading, shopping, cooking, etc. Focusing only on symptoms and medication depersonalises the individual and prevents the development of a trusting relationship with professionals which, in turn, may delay recovery (Case Example 12.2).

Case Example 12.2

On the second evening in hospital a compassionate nurse finally told me what I needed to know.... I was grateful to her for reassuring me; for telling me I would be OK. For explaining it was only a temporary situation.

(Raptopolous, 2010:76)

Experiences of people from BME communities

Patients from black and ethnic minority groups, in particular, report poor experiences and are more highly represented in the psychiatric hospital population than other groups (CQC, 2010). Each year between 2005 and 2010, the *Count Me in Census* recorded a profile of people in psychiatric in-patient care. This monitoring device was introduced to reduce the 'institutional discrimination' that had been identified in the mental health services following the death of David 'Rocky' Bennett (DoH, 2003a) and to monitor progress on the experience of patients from Black and Minority Ethnic (BME) communities of mental health services. Unfortunately, the 2010 Census report (CQC, 2010) showed that few changes in the statistics had been achieved over the previous 5 years:

- Admission rates remain higher than average among minority ethnic groups;
- The numbers of detained patients under the Mental Health Act 1983 are higher than average;
- The rates for detained patients who were placed on a community treatment order (CTO) are higher among South Asian and Black groups;
- Seclusion rates are generally higher than average for Black groups.

(CQC, 2010)

In addition to setting up the regular annual census in 2004, the Government also funded a range of initiatives aimed at improving care for BME communities called the Race Equality Programme (DoH, 2003b). In a review of the effectiveness of that programme, Wilson (2009) suggests that the numbers are not the whole story and that statistics are insufficient as a tool to measure quality improvements.

For example, Wilson (2009) cites Fearon *et al.* (2006) whose independent research found higher rates of mental health problems among people from BME communities in all parts of the world and suggested that this is the reason that we see higher numbers of these groups using services. Furthermore, causes such as poverty, housing, unemployment, culture stress and other problems may also contribute to the high number of BME admissions. Wilson (2009) therefore suggests that although the admission rates are important, they are not the whole story in terms of quality.

Building on these arguments the authors would suggest, regardless of the number and nature of admissions, that the quality of service provided to people from BME communities and their experience of psychiatric care remains unsatisfactory in many places. The following example would appear to demonstrate fundamental and obvious issues of poor cultural practice that persist (Case Example 12.3).

Case Example 12.3

Ahmed (21) is a devout Muslim who was brought into a hospital, situated in an area with a large Asian population, under Section 2 in 2011. He asked about somewhere he could pray, but this was not available to him. He could not eat the hospital food, but it was not possible to provide him with an alternative to meet his cultural needs. His sister wanted to bring in food for him, but this was not permitted on the grounds of Health and Safety.

Cultural competence (Transcultural Nursing, 2012) is not simply about providing for religious and dietary needs. Most importantly, it is about finding out from people what their culture means to them in a whole range of ways, which may include enabling them to share experiences of racism or discrimination, exploring beliefs about health and mental health, recognising different ways of experiencing spirituality as well as overcoming language barriers and using interpreters appropriately.

The UK has been a diverse multicultural society now for more than half a century and yet, as a scholar and leader on this subject, Dr. Carlis Douglas, recently asked one of the authors 'Why, in 2012 would people from an Afro-Caribbean background still need to be classed as a "seldom heard group"'? (Douglas, 2012, personal communication with J. Weinstein). Campaigners are determined to 'break the circles of fear' (Sainsbury Centre for Mental Health, 2002) that leads to a revolving door of readmissions for many patients, especially those from BME backgrounds. Partly because of the absence of a culturally competent or respectful approach, people from BME communities tend to avoid mental health services in the early stages of illness because the stories they have heard frighten them. When they are finally forced to encounter the services, they are already very unwell, and the way in which they are treated can often confirm their worst fears. Wilson (2009) in her research states that

> ...*fear as a barrier to service access facing members of Black and minority communities was a recurring theme in the majority of the study reports, with a significant number, including service providers, reporting this* (p. 9).

Cultural incompetence can lead to poor diagnosis, inappropriate treatment and unnecessarily prolonged stays in hospital. It is suggested here that culturally competent care planning which takes into account religion, spirituality, family, community, diet, custom and beliefs will make a significantly positive difference. Learning about the culture and backgrounds of local BME communities can be helpful but relying on this alone may lead to stereotyping and making false assumptions. It is absolutely essential to listen sensitively to the patient (Case Example 12.4).

Case Example 12.4

I am a Black Afro-Caribbean whose parents are from Barbados. I was diagnosed in 1981 with schizophrenia.... Racism is an issue I will come to later but first I want to talk about cultural issues. In any culture it would seem reasonable to expect Psychiatrists to get to know their patient first. But in my experience Psychiatrists often make recommendations about a person before even meeting them. This 'getting to know you' process is even more important if professionals are working with someone from a different culture. They need more time, both to understand the cultural issues that might pertain, and also to build trust with the person who may feel particularly frightened or insecure.

(Greaves, 2010:66)

Another cause of the fear that particularly black community members have of acknowledging mental illness is the lack of understanding and stigma it attracts within their own community. In some languages, there are not even words to use for mental illness, and symptoms are often interpreted in religious, spiritual or even evil or wicked terms and can lead to the person with mental health issues being spurned by the society. Parents and other elders may berate them for being difficult, lazy or uncooperative while friends might try and cheer them up by encouraging them to drink or take drugs. Both these approaches can exacerbate the mental illness and isolate the sufferer (Case Example 12.5).

Case Example 12.5

A young Somali mother has postnatal depression. She is berated by her husband and her mother-in-law for neglecting her household duties and her baby. The family has no understanding of mental illness; her condition deteriorates and she has nowhere to turn for help.

It is therefore vital to raise awareness about mental health within the community, destigmatise it and ensure that there are people within the community who can provide information and support (Case Example 12.6).

Case Example 12.6

Sound Minds won an award for undertaking visits to black community groups and youth groups where they ran workshops to raise awareness of mental health. They took their instruments and enabled people to play music with them.

As part of the Race Equality Programme (DoH, 2003b), a number of mental health services piloted various good practice projects aimed at adapting some of the mental health treatment tools, previously criticised as being Eurocentric, in order to take culture and ethnicity into account.

For example, the *Wellness Recovery Action Plan* (WRAP) (Copeland, 2002) was tailored for patients from BME communities and piloted on a number of sites. WRAPs are a form of user-focused care planning aimed to maximise empowerment and choice for service users, even when they are quite ill or in crisis. In our experience, this approach is not being widely used.

Cognitive Behavioural Therapy (CBT), another commonly used approach, was delivered in a culturally sensitive way for BME communities in a coproduction pilot with the local Improving Access to Psychological Therapies

(IAPT) described by Heiderali (2011): (Case Example 12.7). Coproduction (NEF, 2008) is seen as a progressive development that moves on from mere 'consultation' or 'involvement' to 'broadening and deepening public services so that they are no longer the preserve of professionals or commissioners, but a shared responsibility' (NEF, 2008). Coproduction means that service users are not simply asked for feedback but become equal partners in creating shared ownership and working collaboratively with providers to produce better outcomes. These ideas are developed by the Coproduction Network (see www.coproductionnetwork.co.uk).

Case Example 12.7

Local IAPT providers networked extensively with representatives of BME community and faith groups to explain the value of talking therapies and to find ways of making these more accessible to different groups by using a coproduction approach. Following discussions between BME representatives and Mental Health Trust staff, plans were made to deliver CBT in venues frequented by BME communities to enable people to receive support in an environment where they felt safe and comfortable. The project developed to provide training for representatives of BME communities as therapists, so that the service could be delivered in a relevant language and culture.

(Heiderali, 2011)

Risk assessment and keeping women safe

Risk assessment

Guidance on care planning insists on careful risk assessment. Harrisson (2003) suggests that mental health service users experience increased risk in relation to a number of specific problems including suicide, self injury, neglect, exploitation (physical, financial or sexual) and violence towards others. He recommends that risk assessment and risk management should be part of a plan that is agreed with the service user using 'a collaborative, inter-active, and dynamic, process rather than something that is "done to" the person' (p. 44), and he recommends that all mental health professionals should learn how to work in this way (Case Example 12.8).

Case Example 12.8

Canerows and Plaits is a voluntary organisation that trains people who have experi-enced mental health services to visit patients currently on a psychiatric ward to offer peer support. Volunteers found that patients complained that they are often observed by staff at regular intervals without any prior discussion about why this is happening or mutual agreement about how it should be done.

The use of 'Zoning' has been described for managing resources in Community Mental Health Teams (Ryrie *et al.*, 1997). Building on this, a traffic light model (Ashir & Marlow, 2009) has been developed as a more flexible and simple tool for risk assessment and one that can be shared by all members of a team including service users and their carers. Criteria in relation to an individual service user under the categories of:

Red: urgent intervention needed
Amber: additional monitoring or preventive work required
Green: stable situation.

These can be preagreed as part of the care planning process and used subsequently to ensure clear communication and swift action where required.

Keeping women safe

Even when female patients are actually in hospital, they can still be at significant risk of assault or harassment (NMHDU, 2010). Although women's sleeping and bathroom facilities have been separated in most hospitals, on many wards, women continue to share communal and dining facilities with men in spite of consistently expressing their preferences for fully separate accommodation. In 2011, the *Daily Telegraph* reported that three quarters of women patients were still on mixed wards (Adams, 2011).

A number of NHS Trusts have developed mental health strategies for women in the light of the Equality Act 2010 (HM Government, 2010), which reinforces the legal status of the Gender Equality Duty, but some have yet to meet the requirements (NMHDU, 2010). All mental health and social care organisations have a duty to prepare gender equality policies for staff and services to consult their stakeholders and to monitor the impact of their policies annually. Current priority areas for improvement according to their recent national report (NMHDU, 2010) are:

- health and wellbeing;
- supporting women in their roles as mothers, carers, employees and students;
- safety and freedom from threat of abuse or violence;
- justice and fairness for women who come into contact with the criminal justice system;
- encouraging women to participate and make decisions, ensuring that this includes empowering women from BME communities.

All of these aspects should be carefully considered in the process of developing care plans with individual women and should be evident in the care plan record.

The *Triangle of Care* (*This section has been written with the help of Christine Lewis, a local carer and carers' champion*).

For many years, family members and carers of people with mental health issues have been arguing that they take the major responsibility for the day-to-day care of a person with mental health issues, and yet, when the professionals become involved, carers are often excluded. The *Triangle of Care* (Worthington & Roony, 2010), which was developed with carers, sets out a list of suggestions for changes that would make their lives easier and their caring more effective. These are:

In an emergency, it would be helpful if:

- both my relative and I had a phone number to call if an acute situation were to develop;
- as a carer, I could call the staff, tell them the need was urgent and I would get a quick response;
- when assessing my relative, the worker(s) talked to me as well, so as to get a clear picture of how to help;
- the worker(s) tried to get a good picture of what my son was like when he was well and aspired to help him to return to this.

When providing care in the community, it would be useful if:

- staff gave explanations and offered a choice of options;
- treatments were explained and strategies for managing the medication were given;
- as a carer, I was given the same sort of information, support and coping strategies that are now seen in many inpatient settings;
- I was given information about the right things to do, with staff offering me reassurance when the person I care about became a person I could not recognise.

The *Triangle of Care* and its six elements listed is now being implemented nationally in England.

1. Carers and the essential role they play are identified at first contact or as soon as possible thereafter;
2. Staff are 'carer aware' and trained in carer engagement strategies;
3. Policy and practice protocols: confidentially and sharing information are in place;
4. Defined post(s) responsible for carers are in place;
5. A carer introduction to the service and staff is available, with a relevant range of information across the acute care pathway;
6. A range of carer support services is available;

Implementing the *Triangle of Care* will require a sustained effort to achieve a substantial change in the culture of wards.

Continuity of care planning

If care planning is to be holistic, taking account of the whole person as required by the Recovery approach (Mental Health Providers Forum, 2009), there must be continuity as people move from the community into hospital, while they are on the ward, through discharge and back into the community. The activities that people undertake in hospital should help and support them to return to the community. This is why it is important that hospital staff encourage people to think about their aspirations for the future. For example, if someone is going out to a flat where they will be living alone, they might practice cookery, learn about money management or other relevant skills.

Recognising skills and potential to aid recovery

Many service users have realised their potential to become healers, leaders, artists, mental health workers, writers or actors as just a few examples. When they tell their stories, we usually find that at some stage when they were really low, someone recognised their potential and helped them to recognise it in themselves. This is such an important aspect of care planning for recovery. It is not just about, 'these are your problems – let's find a plan to meet your current needs'. It is about 'what are your hopes for the future? Where would you like to see yourself in five years time? What are your aspirations, your ambitions'? (Case Example 12.9 and Case Example 12.10)

Case Example 12.9

Devon was a professional musician before becoming ill as well as being a leader in his church. As a mental health service user, he was taking part in some summer activities and was approached by an Occupational Therapist (OT) who knew about his music background. She asked him if he would be interested in establishing a mental health music and arts project in a nearby church. Devon's immediate response was 'how can I do that? I am a patient, I am on medication'. But the OT saw his strengths and brought them to his attention, and he realised that despite having a mental health issue, he was still a musician and he still had leadership skills and abilities. The rest is history. He became the founder of one of the most successful user led arts projects called Sound Minds.

Case Example 12.10

Humphrey Greaves (2010), a service user consultant and author, writes about his experience of having had a breakdown while he was at law school. Despite an absolute determination to work and make a contribution, he recalls how he was continuously knocked back by professionals, in particular a psychiatrist who told him that his illness was too incapacitating for work to be an option. However, there were people who gave him the support he needed:

'The key to my being successfully self employed was that those working with me focused on what *I wanted to do* and not what *they thought I should do*. In coaching we call this "following the client's interest". The manager of Opportunities, a support organisation and my employment adviser were particularly good at this' (Greaves, 2010:52). Greaves went on to use his expertise as a service user to support and empower other users.

Planning a return to work

For many service users, undertaking a meaningful role in the mental health system and having their expertise recognised with a payment that does not affect their benefit can increase confidence, develop skills and knowledge and be the start of a path back to full time work. The benefit system (Benefits and Work, 2012) enables between £5 and £25 of earnings to be disregarded depending on circumstances. Devon would like to see service users attached to all the mental health teams in both hospitals and the community because service user-led services are the way forward; we have been through it so we would know. Simpson and House (2003) describe projects involving service users as employees, trainers of mental health service professionals and research interviewers. Where they are involved directly with service users, they focus on engaging them in decisions about their life and care rather than offering therapy. The studies suggest that trained users with quite severe disorders, including schizophrenia and bipolar disorder, can be employed effectively in mental health service provision.

User employees differ from nonuser employees in how they work, and it is suggested that users who have access to this peer support will have better recovery outcomes and fewer hospital admissions. Furthermore, being engaged in a useful activity that recognises and uses their expertise enhances recovery for the user employee themselves (Case Example 12.11).

Case Example 12.11

A user-led Recovery College runs courses on all aspects of mental health and recovery. These courses are open to service users, carers and mental health professionals who are all treated equally in the class room. Service users are involved in all the training programmes, and participation will be part of support planning for recovery.

Personalisation

The stated aims of the personalisation agenda are entirely in harmony with the goals of person-centred care planning in that they purport to change the culture from social worker-led assessment and Council commissioned services to a system that enables service users to have more choice and control over the content and timing of their social care support (DoH, 2008). Instead of having their needs assessed by a professional, users are encouraged to undertake a self-assessment, the outcome of which will inform a calculation of the cost of meeting their needs (In Control, 2011). Service users and carers then decide with the professional on a personalised support plan that will be funded through the personal budget. The intention to move control from the professionals to the service users and carers was spelt out in a Local Authority Circular (DoH, 2008) entitled Transforming Adult Social Care, which required Councils to have the new system in place by 2011.

A small qualitative study undertaken by Kingston University (Weinstein *et al.*, 2012; Weinstein *et al.*, 2013) into the views and experiences of people with mental health issues who had been allocated a personal budget produced findings that reflected those of a much larger national study undertaken by Hatton and Waters (2011). These were that many users were confused about the personal budget and found the process of assessment very complex and bureaucratic. Many users continued to receive either help at home or money to continue to attend a resource centre although there were a significant minority of people who were able to use the money in ways that increased their self esteem and independence. Nevertheless, the hope for return to employment or increased participation in the local community did not materialise in either study: not surprisingly given the level of need required to be eligible for a budget. At the time these studies were undertaken, although Councils were starting to decommission services, participants reported that few alternative services were emerging on which service users might choose to spend their budgets.

Beresford *et al.* (2011), in a study of personalisation undertaken by the Joseph Rowntree Foundation, argue that the implementation of what should be an empowering approach appears to have been overwhelmed by methods and systems. This reflects findings in the Kingston study with respect to traditional assessments being undertaken by social workers on a tick-box basis, complex bureaucratic administration and people being shoed into existing services rather than being invited to explore their hopes and aspirations for recovery.

Beresford *et al.* (2011) argue that the current drive to reduce public expenditure has raised the criteria for eligibility and inhibited early intervention or prevention. This is illustrated in the Kingston's study where focus group participants discussed how local mental health resource centres had previously been accessible to anyone with mental health issues while post personalisation;

only someone qualifying for a budget is able to attend. Service users who would like to continue to access the service must request an assessment, and participants suggested (anecdotally) that some people would not do so because of the bureaucracy. This leads to concerns that some mental health service users in need of social care who previously attended centres will now fall below the radar unless they become acutely ill. Carers in particular are feeling the strain as all the responsibility falls back on them.

The principles of personalisation are excellent in that they put the service user in the driving seat so that an agreed support plan will assist the furtherance of her/his own recovery plan. To encourage people to come forward, there should be much more clear information available, and for those people who remain concerned about the bureaucratic process, there should be access to advocacy. To ensure genuine choice and person-centred planning service, users should have access to a range of options including traditional resource centres, newer more innovative projects and support to access mainstream services.

The Department of Health is currently piloting personal health budgets for people with a mental health issue, and a full evaluation will be published in October 2012. The Department of Health website says that

> In line with how personal budgets have worked in other areas, personal health budgets connect people who use mental health services with health care professionals, to design the support that best meets their needs in a care plan. People with limited capacity can have a personal health budget; this could include a direct payment in health care where a representative manages this on the person's behalf (DoH, 2012).

Conclusions

There has been considerable progress towards holistic, inclusive person-centred planning that empowers service users and supports their carers. However, to a large extent this progress has been aspirational in that it is embedded in care planning guidance and the new system of personalisation while service users themselves are not reaping the benefit in large enough numbers. Complaints about the quality of in-patient care, especially the ongoing dominance of a medical model, the lack of cultural competence among staff, the continued harassment of female patients and the exclusion of carers continue to occur on a regular basis. In the community, the rhetoric of personalisation can be drowned in the sea of paperwork, means testing and the lack of innovation. On the positive side, many of the improvements have been led by service users, and we hope that the continuing empowerment and involvement of service users will ensure that these improvements, now required by good practice documentation, will eventually be implemented in practice by all providers.

References

Abbott, S., Attenborough, J., Cushing, A., Hanrahan, M. & Korszun, A. (2009) Patient-centred care and compulsory admission to hospital: students consider communication skills in mental health care. *The Journal of Mental Health Training, Education and Practice*, **4** (4), 26–34.

Adams, (2011) *Three Quarters of Mental Health In-Patients are on Mixed Sex Wards* [Online]. Available at http://www.telegraph.co.uk/health/healthnews/8429994/34-of-female-mental-health-inpatients-are-on-mixed-sex-wards.html. Accessed on May 4, 2013.

Ashir, M. & Marlowe, K. (2009) A traffic light system for zoning clinical risk in early intervention team. *Faculty of General and Community Psychiatry Newsletter*, **February**, 6–7.

Benefits and Work (2012) *Work and Benefits* [Online]. Available at http://benefitsand work.co.uk/work-62/work-and-benefits. Accessed on May 4, 2013.

Beresford, P., Fleming, J., Glynn, M., *et al.* (2011) *Supporting People: Towards a Person-Centred Approach*. Joseph Rowntree Foundation, York.

Care Quality Commission (CQC) (2010) *Count Me in 2010 Census* [Online]. Available at http://www.cqc.org.uk/sites/default/files/media/documents/count_me_in_2010_final_tagged.pdf. Accessed on May 4, 2013.

Care Services Improvement Partnership, Royal College of Psychiatrists and Social Care Institute for Excellence (CSIP, RCP & SCIE) (2007) *A Common Purpose: Recovery in Future Mental Health Services*. SCIE, London.

Copeland, M.E. (2002) *Wellness Recovery Action Plan*. Peach Press, Dummerston.

Department of Health (DoH) (2003a) *An Independent Inquiry into the Death of David Bennett*. The Stationery Office, London.

Department of Health (2003b) *Delivering Race Equality: A Framework for Action* [Online]. Available at http://webarchive.nationalarchives.gov.uk/+/www.dh.gov.uk/en/Consultations/Closedconsultations/DH_4067441. Accessed on May 4, 2013.

Department of Health (2008) *Transforming Adult Social Care LAC (DH 1)* [Online]. Available at http://webarchive.nationalarchives.gov.uk/20130107105354/http://www.dh.gov.uk/prod_consum_dh/groups/dh_digitalassets/documents/digital asset/dh_082139.pdf. Accessed on March 4, 2013.

Department of Health (2012) *Personal Health Budgets and People Who Use Mental Health Services* [Online]. Available at http://www.personalhealthbudgets.dh.gov.uk/About/faqs/Personalhealthbudgetsandmentalhealth/#item1. Accessed on May 4, 2013.

Fearon, P., Kirkbride, J.B., Morgan, C., *et al.* (2006) Incidence of schizophrenia and other psychoses in ethnic minority groups: results from MRC AESOP study. *Psychological Medicine*, **6** (11), 1541–1550.

Greaves, H. (2010) Circle of one. In: *Mental Health: Service User Involvement and Recovery* (ed. J. Weinstein), pp. 59–72. Jessica Kingsley Publishers, London.

Harrisson, A. (2003) A guide to risk assessment. *Nursing Times*, **99** (9), 44.

Hatton, C. & Waters, J. (2011) *The National Personal Budget Survey: Summary of Main Findings* [Online]. Available at http://www.in-control.org.uk/media/92851/national%20personal%20budget%20survey%20report.pdf. Accessed on May 4, 2013.

Heiderali (2011) *WCEN and the Provider Site Model* [Online]. Available at http://www.haiderali.com/3DCD2020682548679BDE.html; http://www.time.com/time/health/article/0,8599,1863220,00.html#ixzz1aUEpHTXL. Accessed on May 4, 2013.

HM Government (2010) *Equality Act 2010* [Online]. Available at http://www. legislation.gov.uk/ukpga/2010/15/pdfs/ukpga_20100015_en.pdf. Accessed on May 4, 2013.

In Control (2011) *Resource Allocation Systems (RAS)* [Online]. Available at http:// www.in-control.org.uk/support/support-for-organisations/resource-allocation-systems-(ras).aspx. Accessed on May 4, 2013.

Mental Health Providers Forum (2009) *The Recovery Star Model and Cultural Competency* [Online]. Available at http://www.nmhdu.org.uk/silo/files/the-recovery-star-model-and-cultural-competency.pdf. Accessed on May 4, 2013.

National Economics Foundation (NEF) (2008) *Co-Production: A Manifesto for Growing the Core Economy* [Online]. Available at http://www.neweconomics.org/publications/ co-production. Accessed on May 4, 2013.

National Institute for Mental Health in England (NIMHE) (2005) *NIHME Guiding Statement on Recovery*. NIHME, London.

National Mental Health Development Unit (NMHDU) (2010) *Working towards Women's Well-Being: Unfinished Business* [Online]. Available at http://www.mind. org.uk/help/people_groups_and_communities/women_and_mental_health#_ edn111. Accessed on May 4, 2013.

Raptopolous, A. (2010) Becoming an expert by experience. In: *Mental Health: Service User Involvement and Recovery* (ed. J. Weinstein), pp. 77–87. Jessica Kingsley Publishers, London.

Ryrie, I., Hellard, L., Kearns, C., Robinson, D., Pathmanathan, I. & O'Sullivan, D. (1997) Zoning: a system for managing case work and targeting resources in community mental health teams. *Journal of Mental Health*, **5**, 515–523.

Sainsbury Centre for Mental Health (2002) *Breaking the Circles of Fear: A Review of the Relationship between Mental Health Services and African and Caribbean Communities* [Online]. Available at http://www.centreformentalhealth.org.uk/pdfs/breaking_ the_circles_of_fear.pdf. Accessed on May 4, 2013.

Shepherd, G., Boardman, J. & Slade, M. (2008) *Making Recovery a Reality (Sainsbury Centre for Mental Health)* [Online]. Available at http://psychminded.co.uk/news/ news2008/march08/Making_recovery_a_reality_policy_paper.pdf. Accessed on May 4, 2013.

Simpson, E.L. & House, A.O. (2003) User and carer involvement in mental health services: from rhetoric to science. *British Journal of Psychiatry*, **183**, 89–91.

Stoddart, Y. (2009) *An Acute Care Declaration: Working together to Improve Acute Mental Health Care* [Online]. Available at http://www.nhsconfed.org/Documents/ Yvonne%20Stoddart.pdf. Accessed on May 4, 2013.

Transcultural Nursing (2012) *Cultural Competence* [Online]. Available at http://www. culturediversity.org/cultcomp.htm. Accessed on May 4, 2013.

Weinstein, J. (2010) *Mental Health: Service User Involvement and Recovery*. Jessica Kingsley Publishers, London.

Weinstein, J., Ellison, S., Hood, R. & Jones, R. (2013) Experiences of first tranche older and mental health personal budget users. *Practice*, (In Press).

Weinstein, J., Ellison, S., Hood, R. & Jones, R. (2012) *Evaluating the experience of older people and people with mental health issues of being assessed for and receiving a Personal Budget in Wandsworth. Kingston University, Wandsworth Council, South London and*

St. George's Mental Health Trust and Wandsworth Link [Online]. Available at www. wandsworthlink.org. Accessed on May 6, 2013.

Wilson, M. (2009) *Delivering Race Equality A Review* [Online]. Available at http:// www.nmhdu.org.uk/silo/files/delivering-race-equality-in-mental-health-care-a-review.pdf. Accessed on May 4, 2013.

Worthington, A. & Rooney, P. (2010) *The Triangle of Care: Carers Included: A Guide to Best Practice in Acute Mental Health Care (National Mental Health Development Unit and the Princess Royal Trust for Carers)* [Online]. Available at http://static.carers.org/files/caretriangle-web-5250.pdf. Accessed on May 4, 2013.

Chapter 13

Recovery-Orientated Practice in Education

Mike Fleet

Teesside University, UK

Introduction

In contemporary mental health care, the concept of 'Recovery' is coming to the fore increasingly (Deegan, 1997; Heather, 2002; Turner, 2002; Romme *et al.*, 2009). In order to consider recovery education, it is important to consider what recovery means. However, one of the difficulties with this concept is that 'recovery' has many different interpretations. In the literal sense, it means restoration and revival, which could be misconstrued as a restoration of preillness function and a retrieval of one's preillness life.

As Shepherd *et al.* (2008) state, the core of recovery

> *...is a set of values about a person's right to build a meaningful life for themselves, with or without the continuing presence of mental health symptoms. Recovery is based on ideas of self-determination and self-management. It emphasises the importance of 'hope' in sustaining motivation and supporting expectations of an individually fulfilled life* (p. 1).

However, nurse education has not necessarily encouraged the development of ways of thinking that embrace this core.

Since the latter end of the last century, mental health nurse training has neglected to some degree the impact of the nurse. In the 1980s, mental health nurse training involved, largely, a focus on the sociological aspects of care. Beginning with the change of curricula effected by Project 2000 (UKCC, 1986), this element has become diluted and poorly understood, especially with respect to interpersonal skills (Bradshaw, 2001). The 1982 syllabus for mental health nursing (Department of Health and Social Security, 1979) put the emphasis on social interaction. Curricula since the '1982' have failed to

Care Planning in Mental Health: Promoting Recovery, Second Edition.
Edited by Angela Hall, Michael Wren and Stephan D. Kirby.
© 2013 John Wiley & Sons, Ltd. Published 2013 by John Wiley & Sons, Ltd.

emphasise this type of sociological understanding and mindset (Handsley & Stocks, 2009). This is an omission that needs to be rectified. As Ahern and Fisher (2001) and Took (2002) found, recovery must be considered in its social context.

The dominant theme from the service provision agenda considers recovery in terms of judging the outcomes of symptom severity. The UK mental health policy is increasingly outcome-focused (Holloway, 2002). Outcomes are stated in terms of measurable objectives of symptom severity. Provider definitions include 'full symptom remission, full or part time work/education, independent living without supervision by informal carers...sustained for a period of two years' (Liberman *et al.*, 2002:270).

This definition appears to be more a striving for 'maintenance' in terms of mental health symptomatology rather than a recovery of one's life. May (2000) noted the emphasis of mental health services upon maintenance as being contrary to service user concepts of recovery. In addition, Padilla (2001) notes that the symptoms to be removed are, from the service user's point of view, meaningful. Recovery is not about a cure from symptoms (Deegan, 1993) although it is frequently referred to as such (Roberts & Wolfson, 2004).

One accepted definition of recovery is attributed to Anthony (1993)

Recovery...is a way of living a satisfying, hopeful and contributing life even with limitations caused by the illness. Recovery involves the development of new meaning and purpose in one's life as one grows beyond the catastrophic effects of mental illness (p. 21).

Bradstreet and Connor (2005) and Mayers (2000) write of recovery as reclaiming a satisfying and meaningful life. This meaningful life is being able to live with, rather than despite, psychosis (Martyn, 2002; Roberts & Wolfson, 2004).

Challenges to implementing recovery in education

Changing nurses' concepts of recovery from 'maintenance' to acceptance of recovery as a journey has many implications. Boardman and Shepherd (2009) provide a summary of these implications (see Box 13.1). While initially aimed at service provider organisation, these challenges are faced equally in nurse education. In order to meet these challenges, the first and foremost issue is that of creating the 'culture'.

The essence of this cultural change must be that of 'hope'. For Repper and Perkins (2003), hope inspiring relationships value the person in the here-and-now, believing in their worth, with a confidence in the person's skills, abilities and potential. These concepts can be demonstrated by listening to the person, while exploring actively, and believing in the person's experiences as authentic for that person. However, these can appear as purely tokenistic if they are not built into a partnership that tolerates uncertainty about the

Box 13.1   Ten key organisational challenges.

1. Changing the nature of day-to-day interactions and the quality of experience;
2. Delivering comprehensive, service user-led education and training programmes;
3. Establishing a 'Recovery Education Centre' to drive the programmes forward;
4. Ensuring organisational commitment, creating the 'culture';
5. Increasing 'personalisation' and choice;
6. Changing the way we approach risk assessment and management;
7. Redefining service user involvement;
8. Transforming the workforce;
9. Supporting staff in their recovery journey;
10. Increasing opportunities for building a life 'beyond illness'.

(Boardman & Shepherd, 2009:1)

future. These qualities were echoed by the work on recovery competencies for mental health professionals by the Scottish Recovery Network (Schinkel & Dorrer, 2007). The challenges, and how these can be met, in the education arena will now be discussed.

The quality of experience for both nurse and service user

The desire for professionals to relate to people on a human basis rather than a professional one is echoed in numerous studies (Brown & Kandirikirira, 2007:79).

For recovery to be the essence of twenty-first century mental health services, an essential change in the nature of interaction between nurses and service users is required. Every interaction should reflect and promote recovery principles and values (see Box 13.2). Interactions should validate hope, increase the service user's personal control, acknowledge their expertise, reduce power imbalances and promote opportunity for a life 'beyond mental illness'. The majority of authors write of the need for hope to be able to lead a meaningful life (Wimberley & Peters, 2003; Kelly & Gamble, 2005). Belief in the ability to recover is, for Ahern and Fisher (2001), instrumental to its achievement; belief in oneself is fundamental (Chamberlin, 1997).

The day-to-day interactions between service user and nurse are the cornerstone of mental health care provision. From the beginning of mental health nursing, theorists, such as Hildegard Peplau, have examined and explored the therapeutic relationship (Fleet, 2004). Peplau (1988) defined nursing as '...an interpersonal therapeutic process – a relationship between an individual that is in need of services and a nurse trained to recognise and respond to the need for help' (p. 14). Recovery can be incorporated into this relationship when it is viewed in terms of a partnership. A partnership based

Box 13.2 The principles of recovery.

---

1. Recovery is about building a meaningful and satisfying life, as defined by the person themselves, whether or not there are ongoing or recurring symptoms or problems;
2. Recovery represents a movement away from pathology, illness and symptoms to health, strengths and wellness;
3. Hope is central to recovery and can be enhanced by each person seeing how they can have more active control over their lives ('agency') and by seeing how others have found a way forward;
4. Self-management is encouraged and facilitated. The processes of self-management are similar, but what works may be very different for each individual. There is no 'one size fits all';
5. The helping relationship between clinicians and service users moves away from being expert/patient to being 'coaches' or 'partners' on a journey of discovery. Clinicians are there to be 'on tap, not on top';
6. People do not recover in isolation. Recovery is closely associated with social inclusion and being able to take on meaningful and satisfying social roles within local communities, rather than in segregated services;
7. Recovery is about discovering – or rediscovering – a sense of personal identity, separate from illness or disability;
8. The language used and the stories and meanings that are constructed have great significance as mediators of the recovery process. These shared meanings either support a sense of hope and possibility or invite pessimism and chronicity;
9. The development of recovery-based services emphasises the personal qualities of staff as much as their formal qualifications. It seeks to cultivate their capacity for hope, creativity, care, compassion, realism and resilience;
10. Family and other supporters are often crucial to recovery, and they should be included as partners wherever possible. However, peer support is central for many people in their recovery.

(Shepherd *et al.*, 2008)

on '...the negotiated sharing of power between...partners (who) agree to be involved as active participants in the process of mutually determining goals and actions that promote health and well-being' (Courtney *et al.*, 1996:181).

Partnership as an alliance contributes to successful outcomes for service users (Al-Darmaki & Kivlighan, 1993; Connors *et al.*, 1997; Kivlighan & Shaughnessy, 2000). With respect to recovery, this partnership should be developed and maintained as one 'that is collaborative, as opposed to giving lip service to the concept' (Fleet, 2005:129). Unfortunately, validation of 'hope' is not necessarily characteristic of current practice. May (2001a) writes of the hopelessness resulting from healthcare workers' use of negative clinical jargon, and Bracken and Thomas (2004) described this as 'condemning'. Rogers (1995) considers that this condemnation can lead to damaging self-fulfilling prophecies stating: 'when people are told they are worthless, they believe it. By the same token, tell people they are valuable members of society – at least potentially so – and that is what they will believe' (p. 8).

The overarching message of hope from the literature is that the restoration of a meaningful life is possible (Deegan, 1988; Stocks, 1995; Anthony, 2000).

A key to this recovery is the belief of service users in this possibility (Anthony, 2000), and hope should be the core to all mental health and recovery (Turner & Frak, 2001; Bracken & Thomas, 2004). As Leete (1989) commented:

> *Having some hope is crucial to recovery; none of us would strive if we believed it a futile effort.... I believe that if we confront our illnesses with courage and struggle with our symptoms persistently, we can overcome our handicaps to live independently, learn skills, and contribute to society, the society that has traditionally abandoned us* (p. 32).

Preregistration nursing curricula have not emphasised the type of sociological understanding and self-awareness necessary for the recovery mindset (Handsley & Stocks, 2009). As Forrest *et al.* (2000) found, 'the most important thing that nurses can do is abandon their training' (p. 53). The challenge is to establish the recovery-orientated mindset in preregistration curricula, while acknowledging and ameliorating the theory/practice gap.

Shepherd *et al.* (2008) indicate the 10 tips for recovery-focused practice (see Box 13.3). The issue for mental health nurse education is to develop in the student the critical thinking required to engage with these tips. Reflection skills can be, and are, taught to nursing students. There are three levels of

Box 13.3   Top 10 tips for recovery-orientated practice.

After each interaction, ask yourself did I...

1. actively listen to help the person make sense of their mental health problems?
2. help the person identify and prioritise their personal goals for recovery – not my professional goals?
3. demonstrate a belief in the person's existing strengths and resources in relation to the pursuit of these goals?
4. identify examples from my own 'lived experience' or that of other service users, which inspires and validates their hopes?
5. pay particular attention to the importance of goals that take the person out of the 'sick role' and enable them actively to contribute to the lives of others?
6. identify nonmental health resources – friends, contacts and organisations – relevant to the achievement of their goals?
7. encourage self-management of mental health problems (by providing information, reinforcing existing coping strategies, etc.)?
8. discuss what the person wants in terms of therapeutic interventions, for example, psychological treatments, alternative therapies and joint crisis planning, respecting their wishes wherever possible?
9. behave at all times so as to convey an attitude of respect for the person and a desire for an equal partnership in working together, indicating a willingness to 'go the extra mile'?
10. while accepting that the future is uncertain and setbacks will happen, continue to express support for the possibility of achieving these self-defined goals – maintaining hope and positive expectations?

(Shepherd *et al.*, 2008:9)

reflection; reflection-on-action, reflection-in-action and critical reflection. Reflection-on-action involves returning-in-thought to one's past events. Its aim is to acknowledge one's strengths, developing greater effective future action (Somerville & Keeling, 2004). However, the focus is often on the more negative aspects of behaviour (Revans, 1998; Grant & Greene, 2001).

The higher level skill of reflection-in-action is concerned with 'on-the-spot', conscious evaluation. It is the hallmark of the experienced professional (Somerville & Keeling, 2004). However, critical reflection (Collins, 1991; Millar, 1991; Brookfield, 1995; Bright, 1996) concerns itself with uncovering one's assumptions about oneself, other people and the environment. This is a skill that can be developed in the nascent nurse. We all have personal 'maps' of our world (Schön, 1983), helping us to make sense of our environment. Critical reflection helps uncover the assumptions, beliefs and values underpinning these maps. To facilitate critical reflection, and to bridge the theory/practice gap, critical incident analysis offers some useful tools (Fivars, 1980).

Bridging the theory/practice gap, Odro *et al.* (2010) suggest the use of small group supervision with the facilitation of academic tutors and clinicians. This innovation provides time for students to discuss their clinical experience and performance, thereby aiming to increase their understanding of professional issues. The outcome of Odro *et al.*'s work was the vast majority of participants reported making better links of their learning of theory with their practice. Participants also reported increasing self-awareness and having increasing knowledge, understanding and awareness of professional expectations. However, Odro *et al.* (2010) worked on the basis of developing 'professional' competence, whereas recovery-orientated practice has its focus on interpersonal competence. This can only be achieved through the agency of the people actually involved.

As Brown and Kandirikirira (2007) indicate, service users wish nurses to be professional rather than behaving 'like a professional'. They emphasise the importance of nurses functioning as 'critical friends': '...someone who believes in you and champions you, who lets you talk and listens to you, who creates a space for you to reflect, and helps you to get things under control, helping you make informed independent decisions at your own pace' (Brown & Kandirikirira, 2007:91). This is commensurate with what Bach (2004) calls a 'professional friendship'.

A professional friendship is not a social relationship or is it a detached professional relationship. As Arnold and Boggs (2004) note, '...professional relationships are controlled alliances that occur within a particular context and are time limited' (p. 80). While DeVito (2002) writes of the friendship relationship as '...an interpersonal relationship between two persons that is mutually productive and is characterised by mutual positive regard' (p. 282). A professional friendship is very similar to DeVito's (2002) description with the addition of Arnold and Boggs' time limitation and context. As Bach and Grant (2009) note, the professional friendship has the mutuality of respect and regard but with a fine line, or boundary, which ensures the professional integrity of the nurse remains intact.

As Charlton *et al.* (2008) highlight, the professional friendship is in accord with the differentiation between biomedical communication and bio-psycho-social communication. They note (Charlton *et al.*, 2008) that bio-psycho-social communication is more service user-centred communication and has a more demonstrable impact on positive outcomes. This nonbiomedical view is important; several studies have shown that a biomedical view of mental illness is associated with more negative attitudes towards, and increased social distancing from, someone who has a mental health illness (Cho & Mak, 1998; Bray, 1999; Read & Law, 1999; Read & Harre, 2001). Critical friendship involves moving away from professionals 'talking at' service users (monologue) to listening and negotiating with service users (dialogue).

This change will have great significance for nurses. Mental health nurses are people first and foremost. The therapeutic relationship is important not only to the service users but to nurses too. Service users can be highly sensitive to both staff feelings about them and staff attitudes towards care (Barrowclough *et al.*, 2001). As Hargie (2006) notes, the feelings generated regarding an interaction need to be balanced with the feelings about what is happening to the self or others. Generally, there is an imbalance between service users' power/voice and that of professionals owing to the power given by society to professionals by virtue of their training and education (Mason & Boutilier, 1996; Nelson *et al.*, 1998).

As Foucault (2003:17) comments, a statement becomes powerful when someone else takes that statement as 'true'. Thus, by accepting the values and views of the service user as legitimate, the mental health nurse is giving that view power. If, as viewed by Samuel and Smith (2005), recovery is in terms of regaining a social identity, then this acceptance of values and views is fundamental. This acceptance is highlighted by Anthony and Crawford (2000) as being an essential component of the therapeutic relationship.

To achieve this acceptance of values and views, healthcare staff need to be aware of their own feelings (Latvala, 2002). Cleary and Edwards (1999) found that service users identify understanding and nonjudgmental attitudes as essential to the caring relationship. Johansson and Lundman (2002) found that service users feel that being respected as individuals is promoted by having responsibility for their own care; being able to participate in making decisions. Being accepted and having one's views valued is part of the journey to promote a higher level of functioning and personal growth (Chadwick, 2002; Repper & Perkins, 2003), reclaiming an equality and recovering from discrimination (Anthony, 1993; Buckingham, 2001; Deegan, 1993).

Higgins and McBennett (2007) make the suggestion that 'recovery is more than an end state but an individual journey that results in an internal change in attitudes and beliefs. Central to this change is the discovery of personal resourcefulness, new meaning and purpose in one's life' (p. 853). Repper and

Perkins (2003) believe that Recovery must be through active participation, the reclaiming of power and control. Stewart and Wheeler (2005) support this sentiment claiming that the recovery journey is undertaken through empowerment.

Empowerment is a psychological process (Manojlovich, 2007), and it should be appreciated from the standpoint of both the service user and the nurse (Kuokkanen & Leino-Kilpi, 2000). The Heideggerian view of power is of power and understanding being equivalent; understanding is the power to grasp one's own possibilities for being within the context of the life–world in which one exists (van Manen, 1977; Heidegger, 1996). Therefore, facilitation of empowerment is the psychological enablement to grasp these possibilities, to consider options, to be able to understand and to undertake the journey towards personal growth (Chadwick, 2002; Repper & Perkins, 2003).

The use of the self is vital to developing recovery-orientated practice. It is essential that the student nurse understands their own personal qualities and how these can aid or hinder the recovery relationship. The majority of people, especially those experiencing mental health issues, value working with nurses who, while maintaining professional boundaries, demonstrate sensitivity, empathy, honesty, integrity and show respect (Schinkel & Dorrer, 2007). The emphasis for service users is not on qualifications; it is more on the individual nurse's interaction with the service user; a reliance on inter-personal expertise rather than technical expertise. As Schinkel and Dorrer (2007) put it:

> ...*the ability to build up respectful relationships with service users, in which the worker has a genuine interest in the person, sees them as an individual, and takes them and their experiences seriously. Only within such a relationship is it possible for trust to be established* (p. 1).

Redefining service user involvement

Bradbury-Jones *et al.* (2008) wrote: 'It is incumbent upon nurses to question the truths that hold sway within nursing and consider whose interests these best serve' (p. 264). There is a need to redefine 'service user involvement'. The phrase implies that one group is 'involving' another. This is not partnership; instead, this reinforces the traditional 'them' and 'us' categories. A more appropriate concern would be to consider how all those involved, and service users are already involved fully could work more effectively together as partners; thus aiming to help the rebuilding of lives in the way that the service user wishes.

Transforming the workforce to deliver service user-led education

Repper and Breeze (2004) reviewed the literature concerned with service user involvement in education, while the Chief Nursing Officer (DoH, 2006) calls for service users to be involved routinely in student nurse recruitment; curriculum planning; the delivery of teaching and the assessment of students. Students should be mentored by service users; thus, providing real-life experiences helping potential professionals to have a more hopeful view of the capabilities of people diagnosed with mental illness (Chamberlin, 2005).

However, there are drawbacks to this initiative. One such being the entitlement of users who have teaching roles to the same pay and status as other teachers is emphasised (Happell *et al.*, 2002; Coldham, 2003). Narula *et al.* (2008) and Babu *et al.* (2008) have both found that the majority of students wanted service users to share their experiences and perspectives and to give feedback about the students' ability, attitudes and skills. However, far fewer students wanted service user involvement in planning teaching programmes or in selection of trainees. Babu *et al.* (2008) found that students expressed anxiety about the involvement of service users in education. Main student concerns include potential 'conflicts of interest'; service users having their own agendas and 'over-empowerment of users'.

Happell *et al.* (2002) found that students disagreed with service users being involved in planning and delivering education. The use of service user teachers has raised issues of appropriate training and standards (Livingston & Cooper, 2004). Appropriate training and support for service users was seen as a key issue (Tew *et al.*, 2004). Targeted training is more important that simply offering a range of training (Minogue *et al.*, 2005). Forrest *et al.* (2000), Bennett and Baikie (2003) and Bailey (2005) highlight the potential challenges and conflicts created by service user inclusion in student nurse assessment; especially if professional and service user views may differ. Research into service user involvement in the training of psychiatrists has highlighted this (Babu *et al.*, 2008; Narula *et al.*, 2008).

Establishing a 'Recovery Education Centre'

There has been a suggestion for the establishment of a 'Recovery Education Centre' each mental health NHS Trust in England (Boardman & Shepherd, 2009). There has even been the development of Recovery Colleges in some areas (such as Nottingham and South West London) (Mental Health Network, 2012). Although staffed and run by service user-educators, each centre is situated within the mental health trust.

Such centres support and educate people with the lived experience of mental health issues, promoting awareness of recovery principles among both staff and other service users. It could be argued that this location of such centres would be counterproductive to promoting recovery, and the location of Recovery Education Centres would be best within the mainstream education facilities, Universities. This would ensure that the training is of a consistently high standard, offering academically accredited courses.

Changing the way we approach risk assessment and management

It is UK Government policy for mental health services to become individualised for each service user who should be included in decision making (DoH, 2003). Risk can be an intrinsic part of living with mental health problems. 'The possibility of risk is an inevitable consequence of empowered people taking decisions about their own lives' (DoH, 2007:8). The main issue in this respect is that

> ...*professionally led approaches to risk assessment and management may... ignore or underplay risks that many service users see as important, such as the disempowering aspects of much mental health provision and the over-emphasis on medication to support individuals experiencing distress* (Langan & Lindow, 2004:7).

Closely linked to the theme of power is that of risk and responsibility; what is power without responsibility? (Brechin *et al.*, 1998). Individuals with mental health problems develop coping strategies to manage their experiences of psychosis (Nelson *et al.*, 1991; Carter *et al.*, 1996; McNally & Goldberg, 1997). Some authors highlight enablement to take risk as important (Romme & Escher, 2000; Martyn, 2002; Romme *et al.*, 2009). While it could be hazardous, risk could, potentially, be a catalyst for change (Rethink, 2005).

Taking risks is not about abdication of responsibility or negligence (Morgan, 2000). Rather risk-taking is concerned with making clinical decision that support a course of action that leads to positive outcomes for the service user. When mental health difficulties are seen as the province of professional experts, attempts to assert one's independence then become an issue of being classed as a 'difficult patient' (Hahn *et al.*, 1996). Coleman (1999) argues that, by explaining experiences from a purely service provider perspective, providers destroy the service user's sense of self. For Coleman, becoming angry owing to such an approach is one way of finding a voice, but service providers interpret this anger as deterioration in mental state.

For some authors, Recovery is concerned with regaining power and control (Repper & Perkins, 2003; Stewart & Wheeler, 2005). The journey to Recovery is a process of empowerment and the gradual transfer of responsibility. The emphasis is on the mental health service user as expert; as Green (2003) notes, service users moving from the role of passive care recipient to that of being the expert owing to their experience. This is an element that needs to be considered in nurse education.

Increasing opportunities for building a life 'beyond illness'

As Roy (1999) considered, human beings are bio-psycho-social beings constantly interacting with an ever-changing environment. Individuals are social animals, having the potential for growth through awareness of self and interaction with others. Accordingly, the theme of social inclusion is dominant within the literature. Being a valued member of society with the opportunity to work provides a better outcome for self-esteem (British Psychological Society, 2000), quality of life (Hope, 2004) and Recovery (Social Exclusion Unit, 2004). This appears to be a tautology: Recovery as a consequence of social inclusion or social inclusion as a consequence of Recovery.

Mental health workers' low expectations of people with mental health problems being able to return to work could be especially hope destroying (Perkins, 2005). One potential result of this could be few people with mental health problems being in work; thus creating a vicious spiral of low expectations leading to low achievement, leading inevitably to even lower expectations. However, low expectations are not necessarily accurate. Rinaldi (2000) found that of people with mental health problems but who were in work, 40% had been 'advised' that they would never be able to work again by a mental health professional.

Increasing 'personalisation' and choice

Striving to achieve a meaningful life implies not only hope but a sense of control. To paraphrase Leete (1989) that by confronting illness with courage, the service user can live an independent life. Thus, it could be said that hope is a result of control, when service users have a belief that health is a result of their own actions (Wallston, 1992). Conversely, the current dominant model promotes the belief that health is a result of external control by healthcare systems. Lack of control over one's own experiences is closely linked to depression (Birchwood *et al.*, 1993). This is supported by the concept of 'locus of control' (Rotter, 1966).

Within psychology, locus of control refers to the perception an individual has of the underlying cause of events in their life. If the outcomes of one's actions are perceived as contingent on what one does, one has an internal control orientation. If the outcomes of one's actions are perceived as contingent on events outside one's control, one has an external control orientation (Zimbardo, 1985). From a psychological perspective, it appears healthier to perceive control over the aspects of life that one has the capability to influence (Mamlin *et al.*, 2001). The journey to recovery could be seen as a movement from a perceived external locus of control to a more internal locus.

An example of the perceived external locus is when Coleman (1999) writes of his anger towards the mental health system destroying a fragile sense of self by labelling psychotic experience as valueless and explaining experiences from a purely biological stance. This attributes the cause of one's feelings, and self-concept, to other agents. The anger that Coleman describes could be related to the concept of hope; as St. Augustine of Hippo commented, 'Hope has two beautiful daughters: their names are anger and courage; anger at the way things are, and courage to see that they do not remain the way they are' (St. Augustine of Hippo cited in Macfee Brown, 1988:136). Thus feeling angry and having the courage to express this in a rigid mental health system could be an outward expression of hope. There is evidence that locus of control *can* change: some educational interventions have produced a shift towards an internal locus of control (Hattie *et al.*, 1997; Hans, 2000). Glover (2002) calls on professionals to have the '...ability to act as holders of hope for those who cannot hold it themselves, as well as having the courage to give it back, is critical to good practice'.

People with a long history of contact with mental health services can become well-versed in describing their deficits; retelling their illness story to successive mental health workers. Thereby instilling a fear of failure for themselves and in the minds of providers. As Repper and Perkins (2003) state, '...people with mental health problems have often experienced many failures, which have eroded their self-esteem. Further failures must therefore be avoided as these would further diminish their confidence' (p. 86). Thus, a barrier to recovery is that of low expectations (Social Exclusion Unit, 2004). Those with experience of mental health problems could be risk-averse owing to the fear of both exacerbating their problems and of meeting stigma and prejudice from the general public. However, just like mental health and wellbeing, recovery is 'everybody's business' (Future Vision Coalition, 2009).

Recovery has been described in terms of regaining social identity as one reintegrates oneself with mainstream opportunities (Samuel & Smith, 2005). This regaining of a social identity could be difficult; as May (2000) asserts, recovering from negative social expectations can be more challenging than recovery from the illness-problems of the psychosis itself. Recovery per se cannot be considered outside of the social context (Ahern & Fisher, 2001; Took, 2002). Recovery from social exclusion, discrimination and stigma are themes expressed by many authors including Anthony (1993), Deegan (1993) and Buckingham (2001).

Service user-authored literature expresses that some people experience a challenge to their concept of self after having experienced serious mental illness. Some service users find the need to redefine their own identity to integrate their experiences of the illness-problems *and* their treatment in the mental health system (Davidson & Strauss, 1992; Altschul & Millet, 2000; Repper & Perkins, 2003; Whitehill, 2003; Roberts & Wolfson, 2004). May (2001b) found that recovery integrates acceptance, understanding and management of the psychotic experience. For some, this may be a positive experience. Chadwick (2002) found that the 'journey to recovery' can promote a higher level of functioning; a journey of personal growth (Repper & Perkins, 2003). Burnet (2005) goes so far as to say that developing a new sense of self aids recovery. Conversely, while changes of attitude and values may enable the service user to experience healing (Kelly & Gamble, 2005), it is important to retain one's identity (Campbell, 2001).

Conclusion

The majority of nursing students do not enter the profession to act as social policemen. They do not want to simply medicate away problems, and they do not want to be oppressors. Unfortunately, this has been a perception for some service users. That era is now passing, and we are at the dawn of recovery.

Recovery is more than a reduction or eradication of symptoms. Recovery is a journey upon which service users and nurses are fellow travellers. As such, nurses have to consider ways in which they can aid the service user on their journey. It is not all about medication and evidence-informed interventions; it is all about the relationship (Bee *et al.*, 2008). The relationship is fundamental, and the rest is simply mechanics. The challenge in nurse education, then, is to establish these practices within nursing curricula.

In order to meet the professional and personal challenges presented by this new dawn, nurse education needs to change. In some ways, this change will be a return to previously valued qualities such as social imagination and self-awareness. In other ways, this change will be to alter the dichotomy mind-set of 'them' and 'us', becoming 'we'.

References

Ahern, L. & Fisher, D. (2001) Recovery at your own pace. *Journal of Psychosocial Nursing and Mental Health Services*, **39**, 22–33.

Al-Darmaki, F. & Kivlighan, D.M. (1993) Congruence in client–counsellor expectations for relationship and the working alliance. *Journal of Counselling Psychology*, **40**, 379–384.

Altschul, A. & Millet, K. (2000) Forward. In: *From the Ashes of Experience: Reflections on Madness, Survival and Growth* (eds P. Barker, P. Campbell & B. Davidson), pp. xi–xv. Whurr Publishers, London.

Anthony, W.A. (1993) Recovery from mental illness: the guiding vision of the mental health service system in the 1990s. *Psychosocial Rehabilitation Journal*, **16**, 11–23.

Anthony, W.A. (2000) A recovery-oriented service system: setting some system level standards. *Psychiatric Rehabilitation Journal*, **24**, 159–168.

Anthony, P. & Crawford, P. (2000) Service user involvement in care planning: the mental health nurses perspective. *Journal of Psychiatric and Mental Health Nursing*, **7**, 425–434.

Arnold, E. & Boggs, K.U. (2004) *Interpersonal Relationships Professional Communications Skills for Nurses*, 5th edn. WB Saunders, Philadelphia.

Babu, K.S., Law-Min, R., Adlam, T. & Banks, V. (2008) Involving service users and carers in psychiatric education: what do trainees think? *Psychiatric Bulletin*, **32**, 28–31.

Bach, S. (2004) *Psychological care in community nursing: a phenomenological investigation*. PhD thesis, University of Manchester.

Bach, S. & Grant, A. (2009) *Communication and Interpersonal Skills for Nurses*. Learning Matters, Exeter.

Bailey, D. (2005) Using an action research approach to involving service users in the assessment of professional competence. *European Journal of Social Work*, **8** (2), 165–179.

Barrowclough, C., Haddock, G., Lowens, I., Connor, A., Pidliswyj, J. & Tracey, N. (2001) Staff expressed emotion and causal attributions for client problems on a low security unit: an exploratory study. *Schizophrenia Bulletin*, **27** (3), 517–526.

Bee, P., Playle, J., Lovell, K., Barnes, P., Gray, R. & Keeley, P. (2008) Service user views and expectations of UK registered mental health nurses: a systematic review of empirical research. *International Journal of Nursing Studies*, **45**, 442–457.

Bennett, L. & Baikie, K. (2003). The client as educator: learning about mental illness through the eyes of the expert. *Nurse Education Today*, **23** (2): 104–111.

Birchwood, M., Mason, R., MacMillan, J.F. & Healy, J. (1993) Depression, demoralisation and control over psychotic illness: a comparison of depressed and non-depressed patients with a chronic psychosis. *Psychological Medicine*, **23**, 387–395.

Boardman, J. & Shepherd, G. (2009) *Implementing Recovery: A new Framework for Organisational Change (Centre for Mental Health)* [Online]. Available at http://www.centreformentalhealth.org.uk/pdfs/implementing_recovery_paper.pdf. Accessed on July 13, 2012

Bracken, P. & Thomas, P. (2004) Hope. *Open Mind*, **130**, 10.

Bradbury- Jones, C., Sambrook, S. & Irvine, F. (2008) Power and empowerment in nursing: a fourth theoretical approach. *Journal of Advanced Nursing*, **62** (2), 258–266.

Bradshaw, A. (2001) Competence and British nursing: a view from history. *Journal of Advanced Nursing*, **9** (3), 321–329.

Bradstreet, S. & Connor, A. (2005) Communities of recovery. *Mental Health Today*, **May**, 22.

Bray, J. (1999) An ethnographic study of psychiatric nursing. *Journal of Psychiatric and Mental Health Nursing*, **6**, 297–305.

Brechin, A., Walmsley, J., Katz, J. & Peace, S. (1998) *Care Matters: Concepts, Practice and Research in Health and Social Care*, Sage, London.

Bright, B. (1996) Reflecting on 'reflective practice.c' *Studies in the Education of Adults*, **28** (2), 162–184.

British Psychological Society (2000) *Recent Advances in Understanding Mental Illness and Psychotic Experiences*, A Report by the British Psychological Society, Division of Clinical Psychology. British Psychological Society, Leicester.

Brookfield, S. (1995) *Becoming a Critically Reflective Teacher*. Jossey-Bass, San Francisco.

Brown, W. & Kandirikirira, N. (2007) *Recovering Mental Health in Scotland. Report on Narrative Investigation of Mental Health Recovery*. Glasgow: Scottish Recovery Network [Online]. Available at www.scottishrecovery.net/content/mediaassets/doc/Methods.pdf. Accessed on May 4, 2013.

Buckingham, C. (2001) Schizophrenia – the biological and social. *Open Mind*, **111**, 11.

Burnet, T. (2005) *Recovery – A Personal Journey* [Online]. Available at http://www.scottishrecovery.net. Accessed on Nov 23, 2005.

Campbell, P. (2001) It's not the real you. *Open Mind*, **111**, 16–17.

Carter, D.M., Mackinnon, A. & Copolov, D.L. (1996) Patients' strategies for coping with auditory hallucinations. *Journal of Nervous Mental Disorder*, **184**, 159–164.

Chadwick, P. (2002) How to become better after psychosis than you were before. *Open Mind*, **115**, 12–13.

Chamberlin, J. (1997) Confessions of a non-compliant patient. *National Empowerment Center Newsletter*. National Empowerment Center, Lawrence.

Chamberlin, J. (2005) User/consumer involvement in mental health service delivery. *Epidemiologia e Psichiatria Sociale*, **14** (1), 10–14.

Charlton, C.R., Dearing, K.S., Berry, J.A. & Johnson, M.J. (2008) Nurse practitioners' communication styles and their impact on patient outcomes. *Journal of the American Academy of Nurse Practitioners*, **20**, 382–388.

Cho, K. & Mak, K. (1998) Attitudes to mental patients among Hong Kong Chinese: a trend over two years. *International Journal of Social Psychiatry*, **44**, 215–224.

Cleary, M. & Edwards, C. (1999) 'Something always comes up': nurse-patient interaction in an acute psychiatric setting. *Journal of Psychiatric and Mental Health Nursing*, **6**, 469–477.

Coldham, T. (2003) Mental health is improved with teaching therapy. *British Medical Journal*, **326**, 1399.

Coleman, R. (1999) *Recovery: An Alien Concept*. Handsell Publishing, Gloucester.

Collins, M. (1991) *Adult Education as Vocation*. Routledge, New York.

Connors, G., Carroll, K., DiClemente, C., Longabaugh, R. & Donovan, D. (1997) The therapeutic alliance and its relationship to alcoholism treatment participation and outcome. *Journal of Counselling and Clinical Psychology*, **65**, 588–598.

Courtney, R., Ballard, E., Fauver, S., Gariota, M. & Holland, L. (1996) The partnership model: working with individuals, families and communities towards a new vision of health. *Public Health Nursing*, **13**, 177–186.

Davidson, L. & Strauss, J.S. (1992) Sense of self in recovery from severe mental illness. *British Journal of Medical Psychology*, **65**, 131–145.

Deegan, P.E. (1988) Recovery: The lived experience of rehabilitation. *Psychiatric Rehabilitation Journal*, **11**, 11–19.

Deegan, P.E. (1993) Recovering our sense of value after being labelled mentally ill. *Journal of Psychosocial Nursing*, **31**, 7–11.

Deegan, P.E. (1997) Recovery and empowerment for people with psychiatric disabilities. *Journal of Social Work and Health Care*, **25**, 11–24.

Department of Health (DoH) (2003) *Building on the Best Choice, Responsiveness and Equity in the NHS*. The Stationery Office, London.

Department of Health (2006) *From Values to Action: the Chief Nursing Officer's Review of Mental Health Nursing*. The Stationery Office, London.

Department of Health (2007) *Independence, Choice and Risk: A Guide to Best Practice in Supported Decision Making*. Department of Health, London.

Department of Health and Social Security (1979) *Report of the Committee of Inquiry into Mental Handicap Nursing and Care (Jay Report) (Cmnd 7468)*, HMSO, London.

DeVito, J.A. (2002) *The Interpersonal Communication Book*, 11th edn. Pearson Education, London.

Fivars, G. (ed.) (1980) *Critical Incident Technique*. American Institutes for Research, Washington, DC.

Fleet, M. (2004) Supporting people and their families during psychopharmacotherapy. In: *Mental Health Nursing: Competencies for Practice* (eds S.D. Kirby, D.A. Hart, D. Cross & G. Mitchell). Palgrave, Basingstoke.

Fleet, M. (2005) Assertive outreach/assertive community treatment. In: *Planning Care in Mental Health Nursing* (ed. R. Tummey). Palgrave, Basingstoke.

Forrest, S., Risk, I., Masters, H. & Brown N. (2000) Mental health service user involvement in nurse education: exploring the issues. *Journal of Psychiatric and Mental Health Nursing*, **7**, 51–57.

Foucault, M. (2003 [1973]) *The Birth of the Clinic: An Archaeology of Medical Perception*, Routledge, London.

Future Vision Coalition (2009) *A Future Vision for Mental Health*. NHS Confederation, London.

Glover, H. (2002) *Developing a recovery platform for mental health service delivery for people with mental illness/distress in England*. A discussion paper. National Institute of Mental Health, London.

Grant, A.M. & Greene, J. (2001) *Coach Yourself: Make Real Change in Your Life*. Momentum Press, London.

Green, J. (2003) *User-Centred Initiatives Guiding Lights – Beyond User Involvement* [Online]. Available at http://www.mentalhealth.org.uk. Accessed on Nov 21, 2005.

Hahn, S.R., Kroenke, K., Spitzer, R.L., *et al.* (1996) The difficult patient: prevalence, psychopathology, and functional impairment. *Journal of General Internal Medicine*, **11**, 1–8.

Handsley, S. & Stocks, S. (2009) Sociology and nursing: role performance in a psychiatric setting. *International Journal of Mental Health Nursing*, **18**, 26–34.

Hans, T. (2000) A meta-analysis of the effects of adventure programme on locus of control. *Journal of Contemporary Psychotherapy*, **30** (1), 33–60.

Happell, B., Pinikahana, J. & Roper, C. (2002) Attitudes of postgraduate nursing students towards consumer participation in mental health services and the role of the consumer academic. *International Journal of Mental Health Nursing*, **11**, 240–250.

Hargie, O. (2006) *The Handbook of Communication Skills*, 3rd edn. Routledge, London.

Hattie, J.A., Marsh, H.W., Neill, J.T. & Richards, G.E. (1997) Adventure education and outward bound: out-of-class experiences that having a lasting effect. *Review of Educational Research*, **67**, 43–87.

Heather, F. (2002) Promotion: a positive way forward for clients with severe and enduring mental health problems living in the community, part 1. *British Journal of Occupational Therapy*, **65**, 551–558.

Heidegger, M. (1996 [1927]) *Being and Time* (Translated by J. Stambaugh). State University of New York Press, Albany.

Higgins, A. & McBennett, P. (2007) The petals of recovery in a mental health context. *British Journal of Nursing*, **16**, 852–856.

Holloway, F. (2002) Outcome measurement in mental health. Welcome to the revolution. *British Journal of Psychiatry*, **181**, 1–2.

Hope, R. (2004) *The Ten Essential Shared Capabilities – A Framework for the Whole of the Mental Health Workforce*. The Stationery Office, London.

Johansson, I.M. & Lundman, B. (2002) Patients' experience of involuntary psychiatric care: good opportunities and great losses. *Journal of Psychiatric and Mental Health Nursing*, **9**, 639–647.

Kelly, M. & Gamble, C. (2005) Exploring the concept of recovery in schizophrenia. *Journal of Psychiatric and Mental Health Nursing*, **12**, 245–251.

Kivlighan, D. & Shaughnessy, P. (2000) Patterns of working alliance development: a typology of client's working alliance ratings. *Journal of Counselling Psychology*, **47**, 362–371.

Kuokkanen, L. & Leino-Kilpi, H. (2000) Power and empowerment in nursing: three theoretical approaches. *Journal of Advanced Nursing*, **31** (1), 235–241.

Langan, J. & Lindow, V. (2004) *Living with Risk. Mental Health Service User Involvement in Risk Assessment and Risk Management*. Policy Press, Bristol.

Latvala, E. (2002) Developing and testing methods for improving patient orientated mental health care. *Journal of Psychiatric and Mental Health Nursing*, **9**, 41–47.

Leete, E. (1989) How I perceive and manage my illness. *Schizophrenia Bulletin*, **8**, 605–609.

Liberman, R.P., Kopelowicz, A., Ventura, J. & Gutkind, D. (2002) Operational criteria and factors related to recovery from schizophrenia. *International Review of Psychiatry*, **14** (4), 256–272.

Livingston, G. & Cooper, C. (2004) User and carer involvement in mental health training. *Advances in Psychiatric Treatment*, **10**, 85–92.

Macfee Brown, R. (1988) *Spirituality and Liberation: Overcoming the Great Fallacy*, Hodder, London.

Mamlin, N., Harris, K.R. & Case, L.P. (2001) A methodological analysis of research on locus of control and learning disabilities: rethinking a common assumption. *Journal of Special Education*, **34** (4), 214–225.

Manojlovich, M. (2007) Power and empowerment in nursing: looking backward to inform the future [Online]. Available from *The Online Journal of Issues in Nursing*, **12** (1), 1–16 at http://nursingworld.org/MainMenuCategories/ANAMarketplace/ ANAPeriodicals/OJIN/TableofContents/Volume122007/No1Jan07/ LookingBackwardtoInformtheFuture.html. Accessed on Oct 31, 2012.

Martyn, D. (2002) *The Experiences and Views of Self Management of People with a Schizophrenia Diagnosis*. Rethink, London.

Mason, R. & Boutilier, M. (1996) The challenge of genuine power sharing in participatory research: the gap between theory and practice. *Canadian Journal of Mental Health*, **15** (2), 145–152.

May, R. (2000) Routes to recovery from psychosis: the roots of a clinical psychologist. *Clinical Psychology Forum*, **146**, 6–10.

May, R. (2001a) *Understanding Psychotic Experience and Working towards Recovery*. Bradford District Community Trust, Bradford.

May, R. (2001b) Crossing the them and us barriers – an insight perspective on user involvement in clinical psychology. *Clinical Psychology Forum*, **150**, 14–17.

Mayers, C. (2000) Quality of life: priorities for people with enduring mental health problems. *British Journal of Occupational Therapy*, **63**, 591–596.

Mental Health Network (2012) *Briefing 244* [Online]. Available at http://www.centre formentalhealth.org.uk/pdfs/MHN_briefing.pdf. Accessed on July 13, 2012.

McNally S.E. & Goldberg J.O. (1997) Natural cognitive coping strategies in schizophrenia. *British Journal of Medical Psychology*, **70**, 159–167.

Millar, C. (1991) Critical reflection for educators of adults: getting a grip on the scripts for professional action. *Studies in Continuing Education*, **13** (1), 15–23.

Minogue, V., Boness, J., Brown, A. & Girdlestone, J. (2005) The impact of service user involvement in research. *International Journal of Health Care Quality Assurance*, **18** (2), 103–112.

Morgan S. (2000) *Clinical Risk Management: a Clinical Tool and Practitioner Manual*. Sainsbury Centre for Mental Health, London.

Narula, A., Furlong, E. & Fung N. K. (2008) Trainees' views on service user and carer involvement in training: a perspective from the West Midlands. *Psychiatric Bulletin*, **32** (5), 197–198.

Nelson, H.E., Thrasher, S. & Barnes, T.R.E. (1991) Practical ways of alleviating auditory hallucinations. *British Medical Journal*, **302**, 327–328.

Nelson, G., Ochocka, J., Griffin, K. & Lord, J. (1998) Nothing about me, without me; participatory action research with self-help/mutual aid organisations for psychiatric consumer/survivors. *American Journal of Community Psychology*, **26**, 881–912.

Odro, A., Clancy, C. & Foster, J. (2010) Bridging the theory–practice gap in student nurse training: an evaluation of a personal and professional development programme. *The Journal of Mental Health Training, Education and Practice*, **5** (2), 4–12.

Padilla, R. (2001) Teaching approaches and occupational therapy psychoeducation. In: *Recovery and Wellness: Models of Hope and Empowerment for People with Mental Illness* (ed. C. Brown), pp. 81–95. The Haworth Press Inc, Binghamton.

Peplau, H. (1988) *Interpersonal Relations in Nursing: A Conceptual Frame of Reference for Psychodynamic Nursing*. Springer Publishing, New York.

Perkins, R. (2005) Is what we offer to patients half acceptable? In: *Bipolar Disorder: Upswing in Research and Treatment* (eds C. McDonald, K. Schulze, R.M. Murray & M. Tohen), Taylor & Francis, Oxford.

Read, J. & Harre, N. (2001) The role of biological and genetic causal beliefs in the stigmatisation of mental patients. *Journal of Mental Health*, **10**, 223–235.

Read, J. & Law, A. (1999) The relationship between causal beliefs and contact with users of mental health services to attitudes to mental illness. *International Journal of Social Psychiatry*, **45**, 216–219.

Repper, J. & Breeze, J. (2004) User and carer involvement in the training and education of health professionals: a review of the literature. *International Journal of Nursing Studies*, **44** (3), 511–519.

Repper, J. & Perkins, R. (2003) *Social Inclusion and Recovery: A Model for Mental Health Practice*. Bailliere Tindall, London.

Rethink (2005) *Recovery – A Brief Introduction to the Recovery Approach* [Online]. Available at http://www.rethink.org/recovery. Accessed on Nov 19, 2005.

Revans, R.W. (1998) *ABC of Action Learning*. Lemos and Crane, London.

Rinaldi, M. (2000) *Insufficient Concern*. Merton Mind, London.

Roberts, G. & Wolfson, P. (2004) The rediscovery of recovery: open to all. *Advances in Psychiatric Treatment*, **10**, 37–48.

Rogers J. (1995) Work is key to recovery. *Psychosocial Rehabilitation Journal*, **18**, 5–10.

Romme, M. & Escher, S. (2000) *Making Sense of Voices: A Guide for Mental Health Professionals Working with Voice-Hearers*. Mind Publications, London.

Romme, M., Escher, S., Dillon, J., Corstens, D. & Morris, M. (2009) *Living with Voices: 50 Stories of Recovery*. PCCS Books, Ross-on-Wye.

Rotter, J.B. (1966) Generalized expectancies for internal versus external control of reinforcements. *Psychological Monographs*, **80** (1), 1–28.

Roy, C. (1999) *The Roy Adaptation Model*. Appleton and Lange, Stamford.

Samuel, G. & Smith, J. (2005) A step up. *Open Mind (Mind News)*, **135**, 3.

Schinkel, M. & Dorrer, N. (2007) *Towards Recovery Competencies in Scotland: The Views of Key Stakeholder Groups* [Online]. Available at www.scottishrecovery.net/content/mediaassets/doc/Towards%20recovery%20competencies.pdf. Accessed on May 4, 2013.

Schön, D.A. (1983) *The Reflective Practitioner: How Professionals Think in Action*. Basic Books, New York.

Shepherd, G., Boardman, J. & Slade, M. (2008) *Making Recovery a Reality*. Sainsbury Centre for Mental Health, London.

Social Exclusion Unit (2004) *Action on Mental Health – A Guide to Promoting Social Inclusion*. The Office of the Deputy Prime Minister, Wetherby.

Somerville, D. & Keeling, J. (2004) A practical approach to promote reflective practice within nursing. *Nursing Times*, **100** (12), 42.

Stewart, L. & Wheeler, K. (2005) Occupation for recovery. *Occupational Therapy News*, **13**, 20.

Stocks, M.L. (1995) In the eye of the beholder. *Psychiatric Rehabilitation Journal*, **19**, 89–91.

Tew, J., Gell, C. & Foster, S. (2004) *Learning from Experience: Involving Service Users and Carers in Mental Health Education and Training*. Mental Health in Higher Education, National Institute for Mental Health in England (West Midlands) Trent Workforce Development Confederation, Nottingham.

Took, M. (2002) Mental breakdown and recovery in the UK. *Journal of Psychiatric and Mental Health Nursing*, **9**, 635–637.

Turner, D. (2002) Mapping the routes to recovery. *Mental Health Today*, **July**, 29–30.

Turner, D. & Frak, D. (2001) *Wild Geese: Recovery in National Schizophrenia Fellowship*. Green Gauge Consultancy and NSF Wales, Powys.

UKCC (1986) *Project 2000: A New Preparation for Practice*. UKCC, London.

van Manen, M. (1977) Linking ways of knowing with ways of being practical. *Curriculum Inquiry*, **6** (3), 205–228.

Wallston, K.A. (1992) Hocus-pocus, the focus isn't strictly on locus: Rotter's social learning theory modified for health. *Cognitive Therapy and Research*, **16**, 183–199.

Whitehill, I. (2003) The concept of recovery. In: *Psychiatric and Mental Health Nursing: The Craft of Caring* (ed. P. Barker), pp. 43–49. Arnold, London.

Wimberley L. & Peters A. (2003) Recovery in acute mental health. *Occupational Therapy News*, **July**, 25.

Zimbardo, P.G. (1985) *Psychology and Life*, 11th edn. Scott Foresman, Glenview.

Chapter 14

The Recovery Journey

Stephan D. Kirby

Teesside University, UK

As a consequence of developing this text, we (the editors) deemed it essential to capture the major themes and concepts so that they could be easily understood and then used by the reader. To this end, it is obvious that a visual representation of 'The Recovery Journey' (as seen by us) would be an ideal tool and a way to understand (visually) this process; this journey as experienced by the person with mental health problems and all their collaborative partners. We do not claim to be innovative in this as there are numerous models of, and including, recovery available in other texts (and mentioned in previous chapters in this text), but this is our variant based on our (underpinning) thinking behind this text as well as the contents of the chapters. The model is an adaptation of Kirby (2001), Kirby and Cross (2002), Kirby in this text (Chapter 11) and Watkins (2001) with influences from Kaplan (1964) (who talks about 'Primary', 'Secondary' and 'Tertiary' phases of a person's mental health career), and hopefully the reader will see how the chapters link and influence this model and how we view (albeit briefly) the road to mental health recovery. As you can see, this has three major domains (which also form the frame for this book): 'Survive'; 'Manage' and 'Thrive'. These then comprise various phases of the recovery process 'Surviving Mental Health Crisis'; 'Reconstruction'; 'Growth'; 'Recovery' and 'Reintegration'. Contained within the model are descriptions of the experiences that the person with mental health problems could (or does) encounter at each phase (Figure 14.1).

Once a person starts to develop and suffer from mental health problems and experiences problems coping with how this impacts on their daily life, they become vulnerable as their existing coping strategies, if indeed they ever had any in the first instance, are no longer effective to help them through this traumatic crisis time. People encounter emotional distress and problems with living within the turmoil especially if their support mechanisms and

Care Planning in Mental Health: Promoting Recovery, Second Edition.
Edited by Angela Hall, Michael Wren and Stephan D. Kirby.
© 2013 John Wiley & Sons, Ltd. Published 2013 by John Wiley & Sons, Ltd.

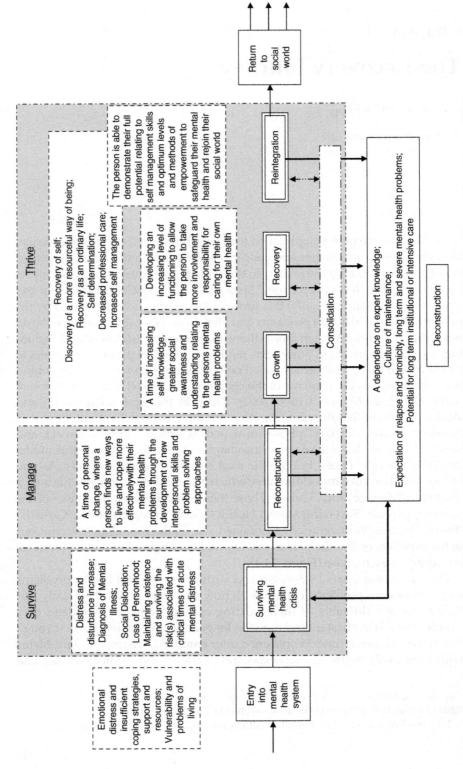

Figure 14.1 The Recovery Journey (Adapted from: Watkins, 2001; Kirby, 2001; Kirby & Cross, 2002 with influences from Kaplan, 1964).

internal and external resources are not sufficiently strong. It is at this point that they reach out for help; or help is offered to them and they enter, via one of various potential routes, the mental health system.

Survive (domain)

Entering the 'Survive' domain, the person is now in a place of crisis; they are in distress and unable to come to terms with or control their mental health problems. They experience social and personal dislocation, they are removed – or remove themselves – from the social network that has, so far, been their support mechanism. There is an acute sense of loss of identity and personhood, and they are unsure who they are in all this – previous social roles and identities are eroded. They do not understand what is happening nor why. Isolation and loneliness increases thus compounding their distress. Simply surviving everyday life is filled with the traumas and crises, they are no longer alive and they are simply existing day to day.

Survive: 'surviving mental health crisis'

At this point, they come into contact with the mental health system and the mental health practitioner, and the therapeutic alliance commences at this stage (see Kirby in this text) and it is at this point that recovery commences. Though at this stage, it could be that the person is unable to make rational and logical decisions about themselves and their care. So it is that the medical model comes into play and the pendulous power swings away from the person and firmly in the hands of the clinical staff. A medical diagnosis and (invariably) mediation are applied and prescribed. In the best interests of the person in crisis, shared decision making takes a back seat and, while they are informed of actions and activities, decisions are made for them until they are in a situation where they are better able to be involved in their care.

Manage (domain): 'reconstruction'

As the person progresses along the road to recovery and the need for the medical model and unilateral decision making diminishes and they can become more involved in their care and engage with (albeit small scale) shared decision making they enter the phase of 'Reconstruction'. This (domain of 'Managing') allows them further opportunities to engage with the causes for and their reactions to their crisis. This then becomes a time of personal change; a change from the dependent, vulnerable person who was in crisis to someone who is finding and starting to learn new ways of living with the effects of and coping more effectively with this debilitating experience through learning and developing new interpersonal skills and problem solving approaches. At this point, the medical approach is not so dominant, it is still present as medication (and maybe other medical interventions) is invariably still required, but it is here that the person joins forces more with the mental health practitioner, and the therapeutic alliance starts to become a working affair. The person has been through a traumatic experience, and it is now the role of the therapeutic alliance to commence to instil existential security for the world had become a very confusing, alien and possibly dangerous place for the person, so he needs to 'find his place' again within it.

Thrive (domain)

Once he has 'Survived' the crisis inducing onset of his mental health problems and 'Managed' the arduous task of developing new skills and approaches to allow him to come to terms with this life changing event, he starts out on the road to recovery. From here, the person enters a phase that will allow him to recover his personhood; his 'self', from the miasma of confusion and alien feelings he has gone through when in the acute, crisis and subacute, reconstruction phases. He enters a period of 'Thriving', and it is here that the sense of 'self' is further (re)developed in his recovery. He continues to discover more resourceful way of being and living. Mental health problems stop being the focus, and recovery becomes the norm and focus for his continued life. It is as he travels through this domain that he reduces his reliance on the mental health professional and becomes more self-managed and self-guided.

It is at this point that the power agenda, moving as it is from the predominantly medical approach and biological model, is being placed with the person and the mental health practitioner as they engage fully in the collaborative shared decision making of the therapeutic alliance. As he progresses through this 'Thrive' domain, it is that the person with the mental health problems starts making the majority of the decisions, though (initially) in collaboration and consultation with his therapeutic partner. Thus, an environment of mutual learning is being developed and taking place, and as such he is being empowered to engage with his mental health problems and learning and developing and growing as he does so.

Thrive: 'growth'

He continues to 'Grow' as an individual and develop new, and/or tap into old, unused, resources for his own mental health problems. The innate expertise that he has comes to the fore and he starts, with the collaboration of the mental health professional; his therapeutic partner, to utilise this expertise to engage with the increased self-knowledge as he develops a greater social, and self, awareness. As the mutual learning between the person and the mental health practitioner develops and grows, so does their understanding relating to the person's mental health problems and the way it effects their life; the precipitating factors, his coping skills and abilities, all creating a foundation for further learning.

Thrive: 'recovery'

This continual discovery of growing and discovering more resourceful ways of living, through the collaborative nature of the therapeutic alliance and recovery ethos, takes the person into a phase whereby he is taking primary involvement and responsibility for his 'Recovery'. This results in, and is a consequence of, an increased level of functioning and involvement, thus taking responsibility for his own mental health and ensuring that he has developed and learned the strategies to care for it in the future. By this juncture, the mental health practitioner is taking a much further back seat, as the person in recovery is now in control of his mental health and the directions his future is going in. He is making more autonomous decisions and is ready to rejoin the social world again.

Thrive: reintegration

In the final stage, where the person, who once suffered from mental health problems, who now is in control of them, who has learnt as well as taught others about this potentially debilitating feature of their life enters the last phase of the model: 'Reintegration'. He (re)joins his social world as an independent person capable of, and willing to, make their own decisions and who has an awareness of his potentials (and limitations), but who is also acutely aware of the factors that caused these mental health problems to arise in the first place and thus has learnt how to deal with these should they arise again. The person is now fully prepared and willing to cut all ties with the mental health practitioner and services.

'Deconstruction'

However, there is a potential 'negative feedback loop' phase; the 'Deconstruction' of the person, which is equitable to Kaplan's (1964) tertiary phase. At any point throughout the 'Manage' and 'Thrive' domains, the person may not progress any further with the recovery process and choose (consciously or subconsciously) to continue to be dependent on expert (invariably medical) knowledge and interventions and prefer an institutionally focused, and flavoured, culture of maintenance and dependence, to one of independence and self-development. The road along, and to, recovery is a frightening prospect for some people, and this may just be too daunting and arduous for them. They may feel that they do not have the internal (or external) resources or support to carry this out effectively. Similarly, they may not feel they are ready to tackle this journey (even with the support of the mental health practitioner within the therapeutic alliance) as they may be in a frame of mind where they expect failure and relapse at every turn, and they are not prepared to go through such disappointment. He may expect not to be able to maintain his progress through the recovery process and may not develop self-learning and management, even in the collaborative therapeutic alliance. Unlike the original tertiary phase (Kaplan, 1964) where it was conjectured that the person would (invariably) spend his time (in this culture of dependence, relapse and chronicity) within the confines of a long-term institution. These days, the person, in the equitable deconstruction phase, he would presumably spend longer in the care of the acute mental health services, be they in-patient or community-based, within a medical framework. At this point, he would be returning (or not actually leaving) the 'Surviving' phase.

'Consolidation'

Also at any stage throughout the recovery process, some form of consolidation may be needed. The person may wish to return to an earlier phase or stay where he is for longer than first expected and thus not progress as expected in order to ensure he has fully understood, developed and absorbed the necessary skills and knowledge and test them out further. Then this is far more preferable to him progressing too far too quickly which may result in his ultimate deconstruction rather than reconstruction and recovery.

References

Kaplan, G. (1964) *Principles of Preventative Psychiatry*. Tavistock, London.

Kirby, S.D. (2001) The development of a conceptual framework of therapeutic alliance in psychiatric (nursing) care delivery. In: *Forensic Mental Health: Working with the Mentally Ill Offender* (eds G. Landsberg & A. Smiley). pp. 25:1–25:8. Civic Research Institute, Kingston.

Kirby, S.D. & Cross, D.J. (2002) Socially constructed narrative intervention: a foundation for therapeutic alliances. In: *Therapeutic Interventions for Forensic Mental Health Nurses* (eds A.M. Kettles, P. Woods & M. Collins). pp. 187–205. Jessica Kingsley Publishers, London.

Watkins, P. (2001) *Mental Health Nursing: The Art of Compassionate Care* Butterworth-Heinemann, London.

Chapter 15

Conclusions: Reflection on the Future (Again)

Stephan D. Kirby, Mike Wren and Angela Hall
Teesside University, UK

A person goes through many phases during his encounters with mental health problems, though as we have seen, growth and self-discovery are always high on the agenda to allow them to travel the road to recovery. Once a person (and their mental health practitioner(s)) have combined forces into a powerful dynamic, the potential is realised and released and allows them to 'change their world'. It is obvious that everybody in mental health crisis, no matter how severe, moderate or mild their personal experiences, also have a large repertoire of resources available to engage with to help them alleviate the source and effects of their distress. What we, as mental health practitioners (in varying degrees of collaboration), need to be doing is encouraging and helping the person to (re)find these resources and retain and maintain them in their struggle through mental health crisis towards meaningful recovery.

> *Recovery is happening and it is here to stay, it is time for all of us to embrace, not just the theory or the concept, but the practice and the reality of recovery* (Coleman, 1999).

This clearly demonstrates the need for recovery to be on every mental health agenda; and at the top of them. We know that interprofessional working and the use of a robust therapeutic alliance which is underpinned by shared decision making, and the necessity to collaborate not separate are essential to the success (or failure) of a person's recovery from mental health problems. We need to continue to break down the boundaries between people with mental health problems and professional groups; boundaries that are inherent within both parties and that are created from within these collegiate constructs and are deemed essential to preserve their uniqueness and identity, but only serve to highlight differences and the power imbalance between them.

Care Planning in Mental Health: Promoting Recovery, Second Edition.
Edited by Angela Hall, Michael Wren and Stephan D. Kirby.
© 2013 John Wiley & Sons, Ltd. Published 2013 by John Wiley & Sons, Ltd.

To consolidate this text, and by way of concluding this journey through mental health recovery from the viewpoint of the contributors: the academics, the people with mental health problems and the clinicians (who sometimes wear a number of these hats at the same time), we leave the reader with 'The principles of recovery' (Davidson, 2008) (as discussed in Box 1.1 Chapter 1). We urge you to think about how each chapter, and each of the themes and concepts; frameworks and models discussed therein pertain to, and fulfil, the requirements of Davidson's principles. By doing so, we hope you will see how each chapter promotes and supports a global 'Recovery Agenda'; the need for recovery to be the principle service model in mental health and how this can be achieved.

- Recovery is about building a meaningful and satisfying life, as defined by the person themselves, whether or not there are ongoing or recurring symptoms or problems.
- Recovery represents a movement away from pathology, illness and symptoms to health, strengths and wellness.
- Hope is central to recovery and can be enhanced by each person seeing how they can have more active control over their lives ('agency') and by seeing how others have found a way forward.
- Self-management is encouraged and facilitated. The processes of self-management are similar, but what works may be very different for each individual. No 'one size fits all'.
- The helping relationship between clinicians and patients moves away from being expert/patient to being 'coaches' or 'partners' on a journey of discovery. Clinicians are there to be 'on tap, not on top'.
- People do not recover in isolation. Recovery is closely associated with social inclusion and being able to take on meaningful and satisfying social roles within local communities, rather than in segregated services.
- Recovery is about discovering – or rediscovering – a sense of personal identity, separate from illness or disability.
- The language used and the stories and meanings that are constructed have great significance as mediators of the recovery process. These shared meanings either support a sense of hope and possibility or invite pessimism and chronicity.
- The development of recovery-based services emphasises the personal qualities of staff as much as their formal qualifications. It seeks to cultivate their capacity for hope, creativity, care, compassion, realism and resilience.
- Family and other supporters are often crucial to recovery, and they should be included as partners wherever possible. However, peer support is central for many people in their recovery.

(Davidson, 2008)

Whether you are a mental health practitioner (irrespective of discipline) or a person with, or caring for a person with, mental health problems, we encourage you to give some consideration also to the Recovery Journey, as proposed in the previous (mini) chapter. We feel that if, in our collaborations and partnerships with people, we are mindful of the phases proposed and the descriptions of the experiences, the potential sign posts; the difficult periods and the potential man-traps along our journey as the person with mental health problems go on the arduous road from mental health crisis to recovery, then maybe, just maybe, we *can* be of real benefit to each other. Maybe by having such an awareness the journey that we will be making together will be less fraught with disaster and be one of learning and hope and empowerment (for all parties) and thus be:

...a deeply personal, unique process of changing one's attitudes, values, feelings, goals, skills and roles. It is a way of living a satisfying, hopeful and contributing life, even with the limitations caused by illness. Recovery involves the development of new meaning and purpose in one's life as one grows beyond the cata-strophic effects of mental illness... (Anthony, 1993:18).

...And in closing

While, as we said in the 'Introduction' chapter, there is no, nor was there ever intended to be, any reference to the process of care planning; the Assess, Plan, Implement and Evaluate (APIE), the chapters all contain issues and factors that are very relevant when 'planning care' with the person with mental health problems and their families and carers. For example, we have been introduced to Essential Lifestyle Planning and Parity of Esteem, and we have seen how, without the necessity to follow the APIE, we can still capture the involvement of the person and those closest to them and still achieve a person-focused, effective and recovery-oriented outcome. We have seen how recovery (as a concept), which is based on the notion of 'a life worth living', can be used as an effective approach to achieving personal goals whilst planning care and how effective person-centred care planning needs to involve people with mental health problems, their families and the communities in all aspects of care planning. The message is obvious: we need to ensure that care planning addresses all aspects of the person's life – and not simply their 'medical condition'. Issues, topics and concepts were also highlighted throughout this text for you to absorb and utilise in your daily practice; issues that strengthen the recovery process; the organisation and delivery of activities that encourage and support recovery. Such things as collaboration caring and communication; shared decision making; mutual learning, and mutual respect; therapeutic alliances and interprofessional working will all make recovery a more meaningful and satisfying experience and process.

We have now arrived at the end of this text and, as we did in the first edition, we would like to leave you with the questions originally posed by Repper and Perkins (2003). Readers may well ask: 'why are you repeating/ leaving with same questions and not specifically answering them'. We feel that, rather than us offering any answers from our own, individual and/or collective, viewpoint, or attempting to summarise the chapters into a salient statement attempting to answer these questions, we would rather you read the chapters in this text and then examine your own services and your own recovery approaches and practices and allow you to answer the questions.

We hope that you will continue to bear these questions in mind and relate them to the relationship(s) you strive to forge with people experiencing mental distress and those closest to them. For the emotional cost of relapse, without hope of recovery, has cost far too many people their livelihoods, family and friends. Especially at a juncture in their lives when they need support and understanding the most to enable them to survive in a world that feels isolating, confusing when humanity from another person or group of people is so sorely needed.

In your pursuit of how you manage your own personal development, we hope you will explore how you could and would apply these questions directly into your own recovery focused, preventative and person-centred approaches (as discussed throughout this text). Supporting people through the myriad of emotional, social, physical and medical characteristics that exemplify how the reclaiming of a person's own sense of recovery is constructed requires emotional intelligence, a clear head and a passion to grow from within. This will enable us to manage both the complexity and the wonders of the human discovery that is fundamental to our own development and that of others.

We feel that your responses to any actions relating to addressing these questions will contribute to the facilitation of the greatest gift you, the individual, your team and organisation can give to people experiencing mental distress (and those closest to them) and that is your time, the resources of other people and a variety of places to release their potential to thrive. We need to guide the person with the mental health problems towards making their own decisions, sharing risks with their community of allies and learning from those circumstances that trigger crisis and relapse. By sharing our collective acknowledgement of what underlying thinking and emotions set old patterns of behaviour in motion and what consequences follow clearly demonstrates the profound realisation that we are all more than the sum of our failures and more than our potential and successes.

We can be reassured to know that in addressing these considerations in response to the questions offered, we will have genuinely tried to do our best for the person experiencing mental distress (and those closest to them).

Importantly, by doing so, we will create a real sense of collegiate and compassionate communication and, by doing so, will encourage closer collaborations. The subsequent coordination of all of our efforts will become focused around the person as core tenets that lay at the heart of facilitating the realisation of longer term life chance opportunities and that the perspectives of the person with mental health problems are, and always should be, first and foremost.

Mental health services, models and operational delivery are changing at a rapid rate of knots. Some are changing to an exclusive recovery focus and approach, while some are incrementally heading down the 'implementing recovery' road, and there are still some services that remain, and either need to, or choose to be, within the medical model. By capturing, in this text, a flavour of the current thoughts and approaches and by presenting a number of the models that underpin and promote recovery within mental health practice, we hope you will be able to take something away and adapt and adopt it into your practice. By doing so, we can continue to ensure that people with mental health problems are given the opportunity to play an equal part in their *own* recovery process and not just continue to be silent and passive recipients of 'enforced' treatments and interventions. It is with this thought in mind that we have chosen to offer the questions again to close this text as we feel that; as it should be, mental health services should not become static, they should be organic and always developing for the benefit of people with mental health problems, their families and carers and the mental health professionals who work in them. *Recovery should NOT be an Alien Concept* (Coleman, 1999) it, and being different, should be the new norm. The future is yours to make this happen and a reality!!!

'How different would services look if their primary focus was to enable people to use and develop their skills, make the most of their assets, and pursue their aspirations?';

'Would this not change, for the better, the experience of using services, and the relationship between workers, and those whom we serve?' (Repper & Perkins, 2003:11).

References

Anthony, W.A. (1993) Recovery from mental illness; the guiding vision of the mental health service system in the 1900s. *Psychosocial Rehabilitation Journal*, **16**, 11–23.

Coleman, R. (1999) *Recovery: An Alien Concept*. Handsell, Gloucester.

Davidson, L. (2008) *Recovery: Concepts and Application*. Devon Recovery Group [Online]. Available at www.scmh.org.uk. Accessed on May 6, 2013.

Repper, J. & Perkins, R. (2003) *Social Inclusion and Recovery: A Model for Mental Health Practice*. Elsevier Health Sciences, Edinburgh.

Index

Care Planning in Mental Health: Promoting Recovery, Second Edition.
Edited by Angela Hall, Michael Wren and Stephan D. Kirby.
© 2013 John Wiley & Sons, Ltd. Published 2013 by John Wiley & Sons, Ltd.